Understanding and
Coping with
Vision Loss

Understanding and Coping with Vision Loss

Terri Cyr, OD

Vision Insight Publications, LLC

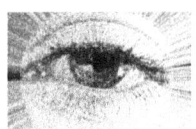

Disclaimer: This book is intended for informational and educational purposes only. It is not intended as a substitute for professional medical advice, diagnosis, or treatment. Readers should consult a qualified healthcare provider regarding any medical condition or treatment decisions. The author and publisher disclaim any liability arising directly or indirectly from the use of the information contained in this book.

Edited by: This manuscript was developed and edited by the author with the assistance of AI-based language tools, including OpenAI's ChatGPT. All final content decisions and editorial judgments were made by the author.

.

ISBN: 978-0-9972453-3-2

Cover and book design by: author, Terri Cyr with the AI assistance of Open AI's ChatGPT

insightintolowvision@gmail.com

Vision Insight Publications, LLC

Connecticut, USA

Dedication

For my husband, David, whose patience and quiet support ("Please don't talk to me while I'm writing.") carried me through the writing of this book.

Acknowledgements

This book was inspired in large part by the many individuals who openly share their experiences with vision loss in online communities, support groups, blogs, and discussion forums. Every day, people connect in these spaces to ask questions, seek understanding, offer encouragement, and share both the challenges and the triumphs that come with changes in vision.

People speak candidly about their fears, frustrations, adaptations, and small victories. They offer practical advice, emotional support, and reassurance to others who may be facing the same uncertain path.

As an optometrist, I have had the privilege of working with many individuals adjusting to vision loss. While clinical knowledge can guide treatment and rehabilitation, it is often the lived experiences of patients and community members that reveal the deeper realities of adapting to life with reduced vision. Listening to these stories—both in the clinic and in online communities—has been a powerful reminder that vision loss is not only a medical condition, but a deeply human experience.

It is these voices—people searching for answers, offering guidance, and supporting one another—who inspired me to write this book. Your willingness to share your personal journeys helps illuminate the challenges of vision loss while also highlighting the resilience, creativity, and determination that so often emerge in the process of adaptation.

To everyone who contributes to these communities: **thank you**. Your openness, courage, and compassion educate, encourage, and inspire far more people than you may ever realize.

And to those who are living with vision loss and searching for answers of your own, I hope the pages of this book offer knowledge, reassurance, and the reminder that you are not alone on this journey.

Table of Contents

Preface

If you have picked up this book, you likely have a personal reason for doing so. Perhaps you are living with vision loss yourself. Perhaps someone you love is struggling to adjust. Or perhaps you are a healthcare professional seeking a deeper understanding of what your patients experience beyond the exam room.

For more than thirty-five years, I have practiced optometry and had the privilege of walking alongside my patients as their vision changed over time. Most of those changes reflect normal aging. But for some, vision loss arrives in ways that are unexpected, progressive, and life-altering. It can threaten far more than eyesight. It can challenge independence, identity, emotional well-being, and one's sense of place in the world.

Over the decades, I have observed something important: while we cannot always control the course of eye disease, the way a person responds to vision loss profoundly influences their ability to function and thrive. Acceptance does not mean giving up. Adjustment does not mean weakness. Adaptation is not surrender. These are acts of resilience.

During my career, I have also witnessed remarkable societal and technological progress. Legislation such as the Americans with Disabilities Act helped establish rights and accessibility protections that were once unimaginable. At the same time, advances in both mainstream and specialized technology—from screen readers and voice assistants to low vision devices—have expanded opportunities for independence, communication, and connection. Yet, despite these advances, the emotional and psychological journey of vision loss remains deeply personal and often misunderstood.

This book explores the many dimensions of living with vision loss—the medical realities, the emotional adjustments, the social challenges, and the practical strategies for daily life. My goal is to help readers understand that what they are experiencing is not unusual, not isolating, and not a personal failing. There is a process to adjustment. There are tools for adaptation. And there is hope.

For those who live with someone who has vision loss—or who care for patients navigating it—I hope this book offers insight into the invisible challenges that often go unspoken. Vision loss is not simply a change in acuity; it can reshape how a person moves through the world.

My wish is that these pages offer clarity, reassurance, and practical guidance. More than that, I hope they affirm that while vision may change, a meaningful and engaged life remains possible.

Terri Cyr

Introduction: What is Low Vision?

Low vision is a visual impairment that cannot be fully corrected with glasses, contact lenses, medication, or surgery, yet still leaves a person with some usable sight. It is not total blindness. Rather, it exists along a broad spectrum — and how it affects each individual depends on many factors, including the type and severity of vision loss, personal goals, lifestyle demands, and the desire for independence.

Vision loss defined as low vision:

- Visual acuity less than 20/40 (6/12) in their better eye, and/or
- Significant loss of visual field (side vision) and/or
- Loss of contrast sensitivity (difficulty distinguishing objects in similar shades of light and dark).

We live in a world built for the fully sighted. The societal standard has long been 20/20 (6/6) visual acuity, and much of contemporary life is structured around that expectation. Our environment depends heavily on the printed word — on signs, screens, labels, instructions, books, menus, text messages, and digital communication. Reading is often the gateway to independence: it enables transportation, employment, leisure activities, social interaction, and access to essential services.

When vision loss interferes with the ability to access this visual world, it can feel as though participation itself has become restricted. The challenge is not simply seeing less — it is navigating a society that assumes you see normally.

In her classic book, **Clinical Low Vision**, *Dr. Eleanor Faye* insightfully described this dilemma of the visually impaired:

"The terms 'sighted' and 'blind' represent groups possessing well-established stereotypes and culturally expected rules of behavior. The position and role of the partially sighted person is much less clear owing to the tremendous range of variability in partially sighted types. Generally, society views them as sighted and expects them to function as such."

Maintaining a meaningful and fulfilling life with low vision depends on a combination of factors: your willingness to adjust, the tools and strategies you learn to use, and the support of family, friends, and community. Acceptance does not mean surrender. It means recognizing what has changed, discovering what remains possible, and building new ways to engage with the world.

Quality of life is not determined solely by visual acuity. It is shaped by resilience, adaptation, and the courage to move forward — even when the path looks different than it once did.

Life with Vision Loss

One foot in the sighted world,

one foot in the blind.

We live with a disability,

but are still able.

We are impaired,

but are still whole.

The rules are made by the fully sighted,

and by those rules we are defined.

We are not less than others,

but are better for meeting the challenge.

We learn to accept,

in order to move forward.

We learn to adjust and adapt,

to live a life fulfilled.   TC

Acceptance, Adjustment, and Adaptation

The key to living well with vision loss lies in three essential steps: acceptance, adjustment, and adaptation. Together, these form a progressive process that empowers you to live your best life, even in the face of new challenges.

Acceptance

Acceptance is often the most difficult step when dealing with a disease or disability. For those with degenerative eye conditions, denial can easily become a coping mechanism. We might make excuses for not seeing well or avoid situations that force us to confront our limitations. But postponing acceptance can lead to social isolation, a loss of confidence, and unresolved grief.

Acceptance Is Not Resignation

People often confuse acceptance with giving up. It's important to clarify that acceptance isn't passive. It doesn't mean you stop seeking treatment, solutions, or hope—it simply means you stop fighting the fact that your vision has changed and start working with your reality instead of against it.

It's an Ongoing Process, not a One-Time Decision

Acceptance doesn't happen all at once. It may come in stages, and feelings of grief or denial can resurface at times, especially if vision continues to decline.

Acknowledging Grief as a Normal Part of Acceptance

Many people don't realize that vision loss often brings with it a grieving process—similar to the stages of grief experienced after any significant loss.

Acceptance means coming to terms with a new chapter in life. It's about acknowledging that, while things may never be the same, you still have the power to shape your future. It begins with asking yourself, *"What am I going to do now?"*—and then taking the first step toward moving forward.

Adjustment

Adjustment follows acceptance and is equally challenging. It requires time, resilience, and a willingness to reset your life.

"I accept that life is different now" becomes a new mantra. Living without "normal" vision often means relying more on others and redefining what independence looks like. Everyday tasks—at school, work, or home—become more time-consuming and may feel more difficult. Adjustment is about learning to navigate these routines in new ways, while acknowledging your limitations and discovering how to work within them.

Several factors influence how someone adjusts to vision loss:

- The age at which vision loss begins,
- the speed and severity of progression,
- living situation, and
- access to financial resources.

These variables can affect both the emotional and practical sides of adjusting to life with low vision.

Factors that Affect the Ability to Cope and Adjust

Coping refers to how we manage the emotional, social, and functional changes brought on by vision loss. These mechanisms often evolve over time and vary depending on the stage and nature of the disease.

- **Sudden vision loss** requires coming to terms with the shock of an abrupt and life-altering change.
- **Gradual vision loss** offers more time to adjust and develop compensatory strategies.
- **Severity of impairment** influences the degree of adaptation needed. Those with profound vision loss may require significant changes in lifestyle, while those with milder impairments may be able to maintain more of their routine.

Living arrangements also play a role in adjustment. Individuals living alone may face greater practical and emotional challenges, while those with family support may benefit from shared responsibilities—or, in some cases, experience added tension.

Financial resources are another key factor. While many state and federal programs offer support, access to advanced tools—such as electronic aids, transportation services, or in-home assistance—can still be limited by cost.

Emotional Challenges

Adjustment also means confronting a range of emotional responses, which may include:

- Grief
- Depression
- Negative self-perception
- Loss of independence

These emotions are valid and expected. Recognizing and addressing them is a vital part of learning to live well with vision loss. It's normal to feel frustrated or overwhelmed. Adjustment is rarely smooth—and setbacks are part of the process.

Once the initial adjustments begin to take shape, the next step is learning how to truly adapt—finding new ways to thrive in daily life.

Adaptation

Adaptation is the process of creating a new "normal" after vision loss by developing skills, strategies, and routines that support independence. Reading, performing daily tasks, and navigating the world all require fresh approaches. Some of these adaptations develop naturally over time, while others benefit from professional guidance and training.

One key resource in this stage is **vision rehabilitation**. Vision rehabilitation services provide specialized training to help individuals maximize their remaining vision and function more independently. Certified low vision therapists, orientation and mobility specialists, and occupational therapists offer hands-on instruction tailored to specific goals—whether that's learning to cook safely, manage medications, use technology, or travel with confidence.

Adaptation also involves incorporating both **optical** and **non-optical aids** into everyday life:

- **Optical aids**: These include tools like prescription glasses, magnifiers, and handheld or spectacle-mounted telescopes designed to enhance residual vision.
- **Non-optical aids**: These can include increased lighting, high-contrast color schemes, large-print materials, tactile markers, and talking devices that replace visual input with audio cues.

Thanks to ongoing technological innovation, adapting to vision loss has never been more achievable. Today's digital tools offer personalized solutions to meet a wide range of needs, such as:

- **Video magnifiers and CCTVs** that enlarge text and images,
- **Accessibility software**, including text-to-speech and speech-to-text programs,
- **Wearable digital magnifiers** for hands-free use, and
- **Smartphone apps** that assist with navigation, object recognition, currency identification, and more.

These resources have opened the door for people with visual impairments to lead fuller, more independent, and better-connected lives.

In the End...

Losing vision may change how you live, but it does not change who you are. Living your best life after vision loss requires a willingness to accept, adjust, and adapt. The journey can be slow and challenging, but the steps you take—and the attitude you choose—will shape your success and sense of purpose.

As my father often said, "You don't know unless you ask." The technologies, resources, and professionals are there to help you—all you have to do is ask.

Be not afraid of going slowly,
Be afraid only of standing still.
— Chinese Proverb

Beyond 20/20: Understanding the Types and Realities of Vision Loss

Blur, loss of contrast sensitivity, light sensitivity, glare, visual field loss, distortion, nystagmus, color vision anomalies, and double vision are types of vision loss. Each of these disorders can cause decreased vision independently, however, there is frequently more than one factor that contributes to vision impairment.

Understanding the Different Types of Vision Loss

Vision loss encompasses a wide range of challenges—from blurriness and sensitivity to light, to more complex issues such as distortion, visual field changes, and difficulty perceiving color. These conditions affect not only how clearly, we see, but also how we function in our daily lives, influencing everything from reading and mobility to recognizing faces or navigating new environments.

What is visual acuity?

Visual acuity refers to the ability to see fine details, typically measured using the familiar eye chart at your doctor's office. While it's an important clinical measure, it represents just one aspect of how we use our vision.

Exploring Visual Function: Beyond Visual Acuity

More nuanced than visual acuity is the concept of **visual function**. Visual function is not as straightforward to measure. It's intriguing that an individual may possess good measured visual acuity, yet encounter difficulties using their eyes in real-life scenarios where lighting is inadequate, or contrast is lacking. On the other hand, someone with very poor measured visual acuity might possess remarkable adaptive visual abilities, allowing them to function effectively despite their impairment.

Visual function goes beyond just the clarity of vision. It encompasses the ability to navigate the complexities of the visual world, from adapting to varying light conditions to discerning objects in low contrast environments.

Types of Vision Loss

Blur

One of the most recognizable forms of vision loss is **blur**. It refers to an area of unclear or unfocused vision in which lines and details appear fuzzy and lack sharpness. Blur can affect both **visual acuity** (the ability to see fine detail) and **visual function** (the ability to use vision effectively in daily life). It may present as a general haziness across the entire visual field or be localized to specific areas.

When blur affects the central part of the retina—the **macula**—it can significantly reduce visual acuity, making tasks like reading, recognizing faces, or driving difficult. In contrast, blur in the peripheral areas of vision may have less impact on acuity but can interfere with spatial awareness, mobility, and navigation.

Adaptive Strategies

People with chronic blur often develop practical strategies to improve function and maintain independence. These may include:

- Using optical aids such as magnifiers for reading or detailed tasks,
- Enhancing lighting to improve contrast and clarity,
- Positioning objects within their clearest field of vision, and
- Relying more heavily on tactile and auditory cues when vision is limited.

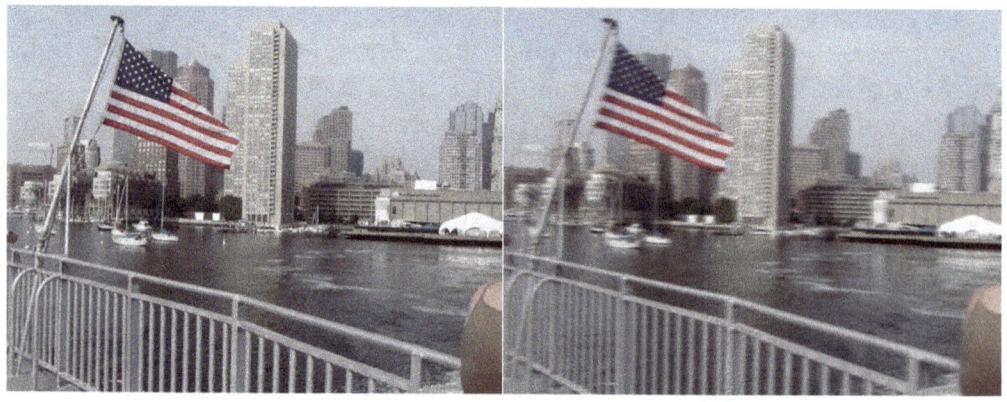

Clear image and generalized blur:

Loss of Contrast Sensitivity

Contrast is what allows objects to stand out from their backgrounds. It refers to the difference in the amount of light reflected by an object compared to its surroundings. The ability of the visual system to detect these differences is known as **contrast sensitivity**.

Contrast sensitivity is a subtle but essential aspect of visual function—and one that is often difficult to describe and not routinely measured during a standard eye exam. Most eye doctors assess visual acuity using high-contrast charts with black letters on a white background. While this method is effective for detecting detail resolution, it does not evaluate how well someone can see in low-contrast or real-world environments.

People with **reduced contrast sensitivity** may still achieve good acuity scores yet struggle significantly in everyday situations. They may have difficulty:

- Adapting to changing light levels (e.g., walking from sunlight into a dim room),
- Recognizing faces or objects in shadow or fog,
- Reading printed materials with poor contrast (such as gray text on off-white paper),
- Navigating dimly lit areas or stairways with minimal color or texture differentiation.

The higher a person's contrast sensitivity, the less light they need to distinguish objects from their background. When contrast sensitivity is impaired, visual function declines—particularly in challenging lighting or environmental conditions.

Adaptive Strategies

Individuals with poor contrast sensitivity can benefit from the following adaptive techniques:

- **Optimal lighting**: Use bright, even, and glare-free illumination.
- **High-contrast materials**: Choose reading materials or labels with black print on white or yellow backgrounds.
- **Tinted lenses or filters**: Special filters can enhance contrast and reduce glare.

- **Illuminated magnifiers**: Combining magnification and light boosts visibility.
- **Environmental modifications**: Use contrasting colors for stairs, countertops, and appliances. Add tactile markers, textures, or color cues to highlight important areas and objects.

FOR NEAR VI
LINE INCREMENTS IN Lo

In one day a full-grown oa
7 tons of water through its

Camel's hair brushes are not mad
They were invented by a man nan

The monkey wrench is named after its inv
blacksmith named Charles Moncke.

A ball of glass will bounce higher than a ball made o
A ball of solid steel will bounce higher than one mad

Panama is the only place in the world where one can see the s
the Atlantic, this is due to the bend in the narrow strip of land

The strongest bone in the body, the thigh bone, is hollow. Ounce for ounce, it
pressure and has more bearing strength than a rod of equal size cast in solid st

Functional Medicine looks deeper—beyond symptoms to the why. Through a thoughtful connection of lifestyle, environment, genetics, and nutrition, we uncover what's driving your health concerns and create a customized plan designed just for you. It's care that supports recovery, fosters prevention, and promotes lifelong wellness. Experience The Pure Path to balance, longevity, and vitality.

High contrast and Low contrast:

Light Sensitivity and Glare

The optimal lighting for visual performance varies depending on the individual and their specific eye condition. While some people benefit from increased illumination, others experience heightened **light sensitivity**, making bright lights or sunlight uncomfortable or even painful.

This sensitivity, known as **photophobia**, is common in individuals with retinal disorders. Due to the way light-sensitive neurons in the retina are wired, those with conditions such as **Stargardt's disease**, **achromatopsia**, or **albinism** may find it difficult to tolerate bright environments. For them, increased light levels can actually reduce, rather than improve, visual performance.

Glare is a related but distinct issue that further complicates vision for many people with visual impairments. Glare occurs when light from a source—or reflected off a surface—is so intense that it overwhelms the visual system, reducing contrast and obscuring surrounding details. While everyone can experience glare in situations like driving toward the setting sun or looking at water on a bright day, individuals with visual impairment are often much more vulnerable to its effects.

Another way glare can impair vision is through **internal reflections** within the eye itself. In a healthy visual system, light travels in a clear, direct path to the light-sensing cells at the back of the eye (the retina). However, any condition that disrupts the optical clarity of the eye's structures can cause **light scatter**. Instead of being sharply focused on the retina, scattered light bounces around inside the eye, producing the phenomenon known as **internal glare**. Damage to the **cornea**, the presence of **lens opacities such as cataracts**, or **vitreous floaters** can all contribute to this internal scattering of light.

Adaptive Strategies

People with light sensitivity and glare-related issues can take proactive steps to improve visual comfort and safety. Helpful strategies include:

- **Wearing tinted or polarized lenses**: These reduce light intensity and glare from reflective surfaces. Specific filters can be selected based on the condition and environment.
- **Using hats with brims or visors**: These provide shade and help control light exposure outdoors.
- **Controlling indoor lighting**: Use adjustable task lighting, avoid bare bulbs, and consider warm-toned or diffused light sources to reduce harsh reflections.
- **Installing glare-reducing window films or blinds**: These limit excessive sunlight indoors while maintaining ambient lighting.

By managing their environment and using specialized tools, individuals with light sensitivity can significantly reduce discomfort and maintain better visual function in bright or reflective settings.

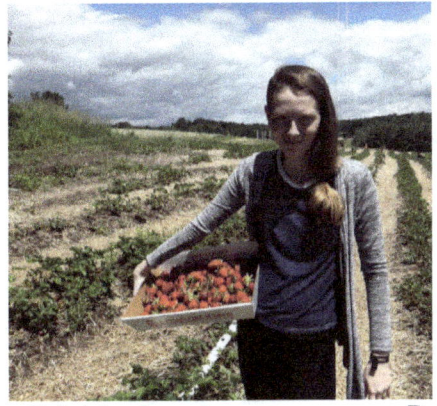
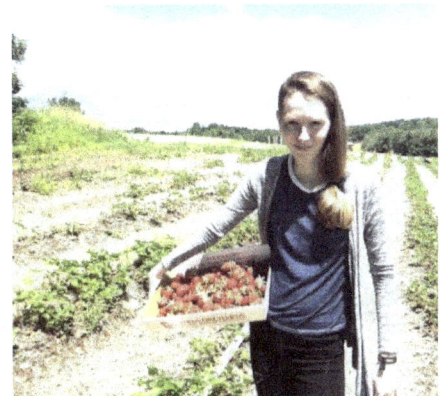

Bright, clear image.   Brightness overpowers visible details

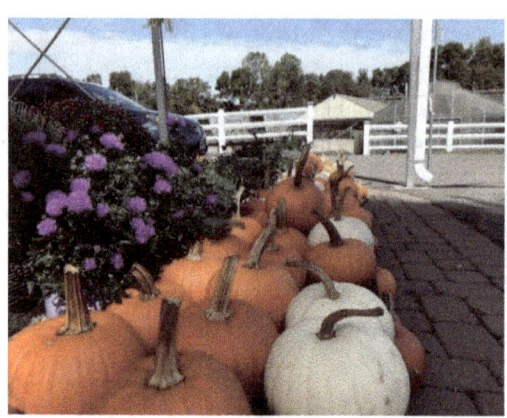 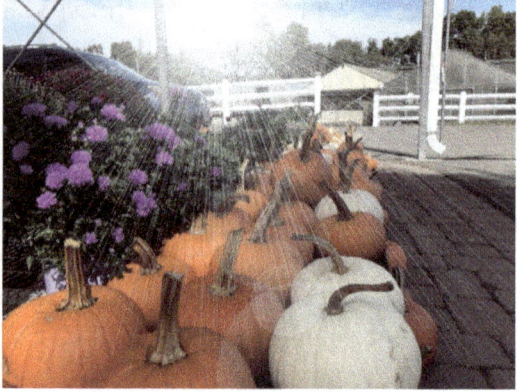

Bright sharp details.   Details obscured by glare.

Visual Field Loss and Scotoma

The visual field encompasses the entire area we can see, including the central macula and the peripheral or "side" visual areas. In people with normal binocular vision, the visual fields from both eyes overlap to provide a wide, panoramic view—spanning approximately 190 degrees horizontally and about 130 degrees vertically. While peripheral vision is less detail-sensitive than central vision, it plays an important role in detecting light and motion, which supports orientation and safe navigation.

Loss of central vision—such as in macular degeneration—results in reduced visual acuity, making tasks like reading, writing, and recognizing faces more difficult. In contrast, loss of peripheral vision compromises **spatial awareness** and mobility, increasing the risk of falls or collisions and making activities like driving or walking through unfamiliar environments more challenging.

Scotomas are blind spots or areas of diminished vision that result from damage to retinal cells. The impact of a scotoma depends on several factors, including its location in the visual field, its size and depth, and whether it occurs in one or both eyes.

Central scotomas are particularly disruptive because they affect the macular region—the part of the retina densely packed with cone cells responsible for sharp central vision. Conditions such as age-related macular degeneration (AMD) and Stargardt disease can cause central scotomas, leading to difficulty with reading, recognizing faces, and performing tasks that require fine detail.

12

However, even when central vision is impaired, individuals can often continue to function visually by learning to use their peripheral vision and adopting adaptive techniques.

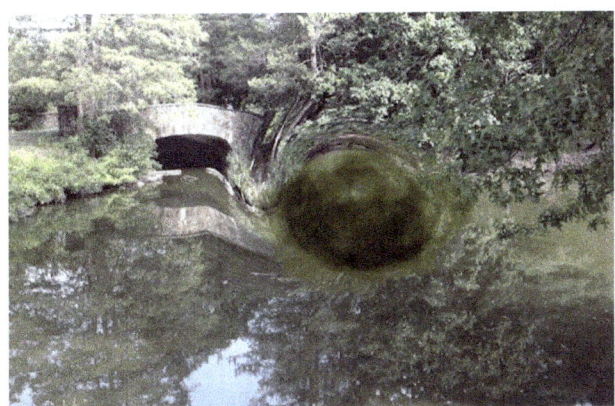

Central vision loss, comparable to how those
with macular degeneration see.

Peripheral field loss refers to vision loss outside the central macular area, affecting the broader retinal regions responsible for side or peripheral vision. This type of loss can occur in patches, in entire quadrants or hemispheres, or as isolated localized defects.

Several conditions can lead to peripheral field loss. **Glaucoma**, a progressive optic nerve disease, is a leading cause. It typically begins with subtle peripheral vision changes that may go unnoticed until the loss becomes more advanced. **Optic neuritis**, often associated with multiple sclerosis or other inflammatory disorders, can also result in peripheral visual field deficits, depending on which fibers of the optic nerve are affected. **Retinitis pigmentosa**, an inherited degenerative retinal disease, is another significant cause. It characteristically produces a gradual constriction of the peripheral visual field, often described as "**tunnel vision**," as the rod photoreceptors responsible for night and side vision progressively deteriorate.

Peripheral field loss can significantly impair a person's ability to move about safely, detect motion, or navigate complex environments. In some cases, individuals may be unaware of the missing visual information, a condition known as **visual neglect** or anosognosia. This makes early detection through visual field testing especially important.

Peripheral field loss. and Visual Field Analysis

Visual field testing is a standard diagnostic tool used in eye care clinics to detect and map areas of visual field loss. This computerized test assesses how well the eye can detect light stimuli at various points in the visual field. The resulting analysis provides a visual representation of any deficits, such as blind spots or areas of reduced sensitivity—illustrating how visual field loss may appear in real-world vision.

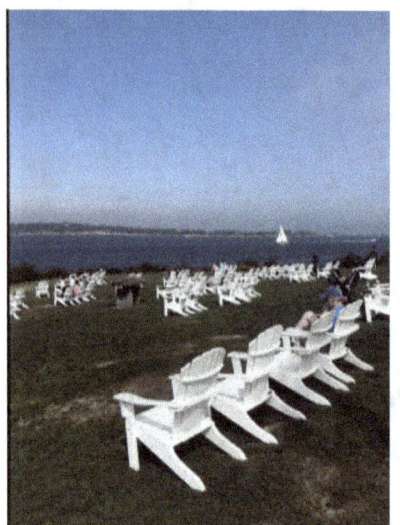 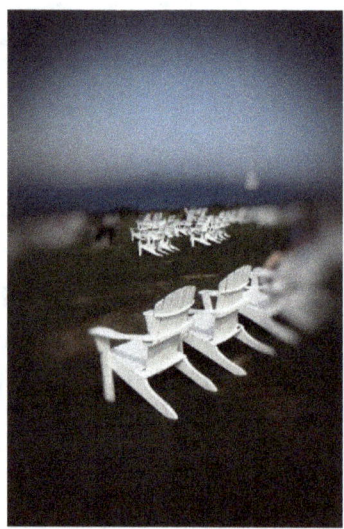

Right image simulates peripheral field loss

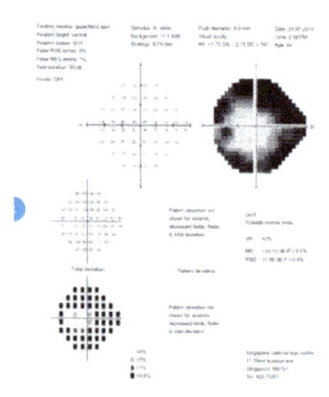 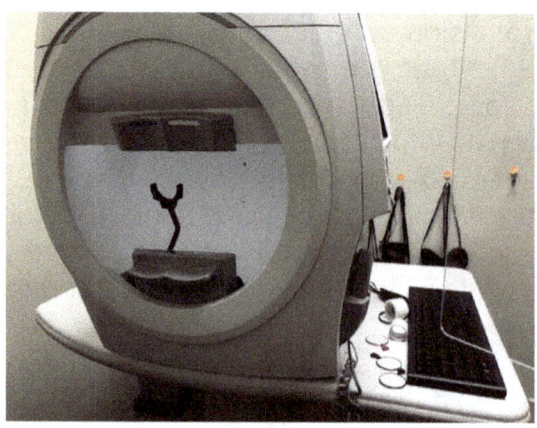

Print out of a visual field analysis, Humphrey Visual Field Analyzer.

Significant areas of vision loss, as identified on the test, can affect daily functioning. Blind spots or large regions of impaired vision can hinder safe navigation, increasing the risk of bumping into unseen objects, missing steps or curbs, or colliding with architectural obstacles. These challenges can be especially disorienting in unfamiliar environments or in low lighting.

Adapting to Visual Field Loss

Although visual field loss presents real challenges, many individuals learn to compensate with training and assistive techniques. Orientation and mobility specialists can teach **scanning** strategies to help detect obstacles in the periphery, while low vision therapists may introduce tools such as **prism glasses** or **visual field expanders**. Even simple adjustments—like improved lighting and high-contrast markings—can enhance safety and independence.

Distortion

Visual distortion is a common phenomenon that often affects the central area of vision, particularly the macula, though it can occur anywhere in the visual field. To understand this effect, imagine the light-sensitive photoreceptor cells in the retina as rows of soldiers standing upright, neatly aligned shoulder to shoulder. When fluid buildup, swelling, or toxic waste products disrupt this orderly arrangement—such as in macular edema or age-related macular degeneration— these cells become disorganized.

The brain interprets this disorganization as visual distortion. Straight lines may appear wavy, the edges of walls might seem to bend or tilt, and printed words can look jumbled or uneven. The severity of distortion varies depending on the cause and extent of retinal disruption, but even mild cases can interfere with everyday tasks like reading, driving, or recognizing faces.

Adaptive Strategies

Understanding the cause of visual distortion is essential, as many underlying conditions—such as macular degeneration, epiretinal membranes, or diabetic macular edema—can be managed or treated. Low vision specialists may recommend magnifiers, contrast enhancement tools, or environmental modifications to help reduce the functional impact of distortion in daily life.

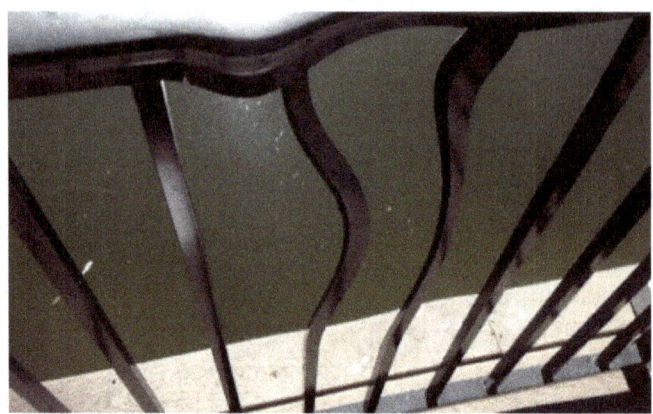

Central vision distortion.

Nystagmus

Nystagmus is a condition characterized by rhythmic, involuntary eye movements that interfere with stable vision. These movements can cause the eyes to appear to "jiggle" or shift continuously—a sensation referred to as *oscillopsia,* in which the visual world seems to move or bounce. Because the eyes cannot maintain steady fixation, individuals often experience blurred or unstable vision.

The direction of these movements can vary—they may occur side to side (horizontal), up and down (vertical), or in circular (rotary) patterns. The size, speed, and frequency of the movements also differ from person to person. Various factors such as fatigue, stress, or emotional excitement can temporarily intensify the movements and their effects on vision.

Adaptive Strategies

While there is no universal cure for nystagmus, several management strategies aim to improve visual function and reduce discomfort. These may include the use of glasses with prisms, contact lenses that help stabilize gaze, or medications in certain cases. Some individuals benefit from surgical procedures to reposition the eye muscles and reduce the severity of the movements. Occupational and low vision therapists can also teach strategies for optimizing lighting, head positioning, and visual tasks to help mitigate the impact of nystagmus in daily life.

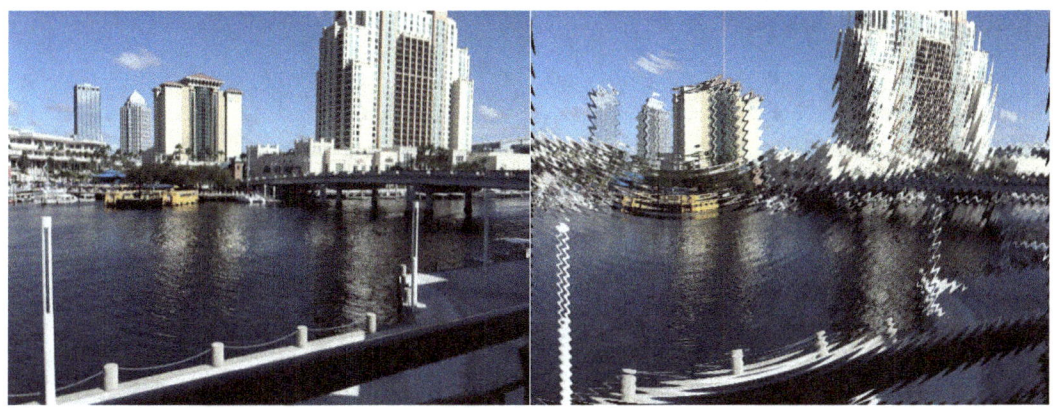

| Clear, stable image | Blur due to the eye movement of nystagmus. |

Color Vision Anomalies

Color deficiencies can arise either as congenital anomalies or as acquired conditions resulting from disease processes.

The term "color blind" is commonly used to describe a congenital color vision deficiency, which affects approximately 8 to 10 percent of the population—predominantly males. However, "color deficiency" or "partial color vision" is more accurate. Individuals with this condition do perceive color, but lack the photopigment sensitivity required to distinguish certain wavelengths of light.

The most common congenital form affects the red-green spectrum, causing red and green hues to appear similar or be easily confused. A rarer type affects the blue-yellow spectrum. Congenital color deficiencies are typically present in both eyes equally and are stable—they do not worsen over time and are not related to disease.

A more severe congenital anomaly is **achromatopsia**, also known as **rod monochromacy**. This rare condition involves a complete or partial absence of all three cone photopigments (red, green, and blue). Individuals with achromatopsia may see the world in shades of gray and often experience additional symptoms such as extreme light sensitivity (photophobia), reduced visual acuity, and nystagmus.

Adaptive Strategies

Specialized "color blind corrective" eyeglass lenses are available for some individuals with red-green deficiencies. These lenses use selective light filtering to enhance contrast and color discrimination, improving functional color perception in daily nativities.

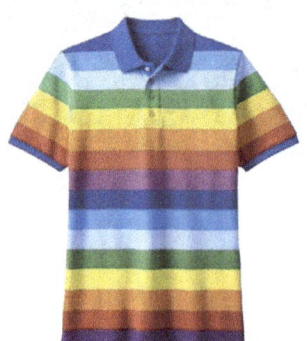

Colorful image.   Red-green color deficiency.

Acquired Color Deficiencies

Acquired color vision loss occurs after birth and is typically associated with disease or injury. Unlike congenital deficiencies, acquired color loss often affects one eye more than the other and may progress over time. It is usually accompanied by other visual symptoms, such as decreased acuity or visual field loss.

Several inherited retinal diseases can lead to changes in color sensitivity as they progress:

- **Best's Vitelliform Dystrophy**
- **Stargardt's Disease** (juvenile macular degeneration)
- **Retinitis Pigmentosa**

Adult-onset conditions can also impact color vision:

- **Diabetes**, **glaucoma**, and **cataracts** may reduce color perception. Cataracts, in particular, act as a yellow filter, dulling and altering the appearance of colors.
- **Optic nerve diseases** such as **optic neuritis** and **optic atrophy** often result in color vision changes.

- *Optic neuritis*, often linked to multiple sclerosis, autoimmune disorders, or infections, leads to inflammation of the optic nerve, reducing visual acuity and making colors appear pale or washed out.
- *Optic atrophy* involves the gradual degeneration of optic nerve fibers, resulting in scotomas, visual field loss, reduced acuity, and diminished color vision. Causes include strokes, hypertension, trauma, or exposure to toxins such as alcohol.

Because acquired color vision changes may indicate underlying disease, a full eye examination is essential when such symptoms arise.

Double Vision

Double vision, or *diplopia*, refers to the perception of two images of a single object. It can present in two distinct forms: **monocular** (in one eye) or **binocular** (in both eyes).

Monocular Diplopia

Monocular double vision occurs when the doubling persists with just one eye open. This can be determined by covering each eye separately—if the double image remains when only one eye is uncovered, the cause is likely monocular.

Causes of monocular diplopia range from benign to more serious. Uncorrected astigmatism is a common cause and can often be resolved with prescription glasses. However, more complex issues such as corneal irregularities (from keratoconus or scarring), lens displacement, cataracts, or trauma to the eye can also result in monocular diplopia.

Binocular Diplopia

Binocular double vision occurs only when both eyes are open. In normal vision, each eye sends an image to the brain, which fuses the two into a single, unified picture. This coordination is made possible by the "yoking" of eye muscles and nerves, which develop in tandem during early life. A helpful analogy is that of a pair of oxen yoked together—moving in the same direction, at the same speed, to maintain alignment.

When this yoking system is disrupted, the eyes may become misaligned, leading to double vision. The duplicated images can appear side-by-side, vertically displaced, or tilted. The severity of the misalignment may vary, from slight ghosting to widely separated images. Double vision may be **transient** (brief), **episodic**, or **permanent**, depending on the underlying cause.

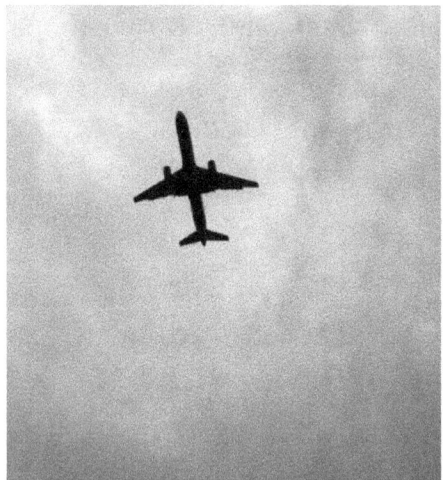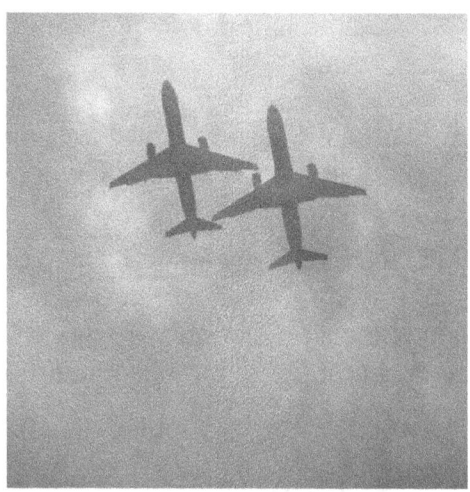

Doubling of an image can overlap or can be distinctly separate.

Numerous neurological and neuromuscular conditions can cause binocular diplopia:

- **Myasthenia gravis**, a disorder affecting nerve-muscle communication, can lead to muscle weakness or paralysis (paresis), including the muscles that control eye movement.
- **Diabetes**, **high blood pressure**, and **strokes** can affect cranial nerves that coordinate eye movements.
- **Tumors**, such as pituitary adenomas or other space-occupying lesions, can compress or damage these nerves.
- **Head trauma** may damage the nerves or eye muscles, or cause muscle entrapment within the orbit, resulting in misalignment and diplopia.

Adaptive Strategies

Anyone experiencing double vision should undergo prompt evaluation by an eye care professional to determine the underlying cause. Depending on the diagnosis, treatment options may include prism glasses, patching, corrective surgery, or management of the associated systemic or neurological condition.

In the End...

Vision impairment is a complex and multifaceted challenge. It involves more than just a reduction in visual acuity—it encompasses a wide range of visual disturbances that collectively contribute to diminished visual function.

Understanding these different aspects and how they interact is essential for developing effective strategies to manage vision loss. Whether addressing blurriness, contrast sensitivity, visual field deficits, color vision anomalies, or double vision, each type of impairment requires individualized assessment and tailored solutions.

By recognizing the unique features and functional impacts of each form of vision loss, individuals, caregivers, and healthcare professionals can collaborate to preserve and enhance visual function. Through early intervention, adaptive strategies, and supportive technologies, it is possible to improve quality of life for those living with visual impairment.

Getting Help When You Have Vision Loss

Low vision services offer a multi-disciplinary approach to assist individuals with subnormal vision in adjusting, and adapting to maintain independence and quality of life. These services encompass a range of professionals including low vision specialists, rehabilitation experts, orientation and mobility specialists, teachers, and counselors.

If you're seeking support for vision loss, these services can provide invaluable assistance tailored to your unique needs.

Who is a low vision patient?

Those who experience permanent vision loss, uncorrectable with eyeglasses or contact lenses, are candidates for specialized low vision services.

Individuals with vision less than 20/40 (6/12) in their better eye (where the other eye is worse) qualify for low vision services. Additionally, those who have experienced a loss of visual field (also known as "side vision") or contrast sensitivity (difficulty distinguishing objects in similar shades of light and dark) can benefit from these services.

Referrals for low vision services are invaluable for individuals' facing challenges with reading, driving, completing daily tasks, mobility, or experiencing emotional difficulties.

Low vision services are not only important for adults but also for children with inherited or acquired vision loss. Children have access to a range of therapies aimed at helping them adjust and adapt to their condition.

Understanding Functional Vision

There is a growing movement to reassess a patient's functional vision <u>not</u> solely based on numerical measurements like visual acuity, degree of field loss, or contrast sensitivity, but on **how these factors affect the individual's daily**

functioning. These assessments are conducted by low vision specialists. While these numbers provide valuable data, they may not fully capture the individual's actual visual experience, which can vary widely among people with vision impairments.

For instance, an individual with a visual acuity of 20/40 might be mildly bothered by the decrease in clarity but find it does not significantly impact their work or hobbies. Conversely, an artist or editor may experience profound despair due to the loss of visual detail at the same acuity level.

Consider someone with glaucoma who has lost a sector of their vision. The extent of impairment will be influenced by the size and location of this visual field loss.

Another example is a person with decreased contrast sensitivity, often due to cataracts. One individual might hardly notice the loss, while another may feel a constant unease due to the perceived dimness in their surroundings. It's possible to have poor contrast sensitivity yet maintain good visual acuity.

Additionally, individuals with conditions like macular degeneration or Stargardt's disease may have complete central vision loss, leading to a "legally blind" classification, however, with appropriate low vision aids and techniques like eccentric fixation, they can function effectively in daily life.

It is how you use your remaining vision determines how you function with vision loss by:

- Compensatory techniques, with and without aids,
- adaptations to surroundings,
- visual skills, like eccentric viewing and scanning,
- add in; use of other senses, like hearing and touch.

Specialists in low vision, rehabilitation, mobility, and counseling conduct comprehensive **functional vision assessments**. These assessments encompass inquiries into how vision loss has impacted various aspects of your life, including daily activities, work, personal needs, and psychological well-being.

The assessment also involves tests to gauge your progress in developing visual compensatory skills and adaptations. The results of these assessments guide the specialists in formulating personalized plans for low vision services tailored to your specific functional vision needs.

24

Common issues identified by individuals with vision loss when seeking a low vision evaluation and rehabilitation services:

1. Difficulty reading and writing.
2. Challenges seeing televisions or electronic screens.
3. Trouble recognizing faces.
4. Struggles with identifying appliance dials.
5. Headaches and eyestrain.
6. Bumping into corners or missing stairs.
7. Persistent sadness or anxiety.
8. Increased social isolation.

Who provides low vision services and where can low vision services be found?

If you're seeking support for vision loss, these services can provide invaluable assistance tailored to your unique needs.

Starting Point: Low Vision Evaluation

Low vision specialists, typically a **licensed optometrist**, who possess a deep understanding of the disease process and prognosis due to their medical training. They are well-versed in functional vision loss and are aware of its limitations. These specialists have encountered individuals with similar visual challenges before, so they will not perceive age or debilitation as obstacles. Their primary objective is to assist in maximizing your visual potential and guide you through the adjustment and adaptation process.

Here are the reasons to get a low vision evaluation;
1. To Advocate for Yourself;
The low vision evaluation is your opportunity to interact with someone who understands your concerns can answer your questions.

2. Introduction to Visual Aids and Techniques;
The benefit of seeing a specialist is that he/she, because of knowledge and experience, can guide you in selecting the aids that would be helpful to you.

3. Education and Counseling

Prepare yourself for a very honest discussion about your impairment and options for rehabilitation. The discussion should be tailored to you and your needs.

4. Appropriate Referrals;

They typically are familiar with state and local agencies for educational services, social services, psychological counseling, and eligibility requirements. They may also know of support groups for those with similar vision losses.

The low vision evaluation with a low vision optometrist commences with a comprehensive history and a series of questions to discern your concerns and requirements. The aim is to enhance your abilities in education, work, self-help, and recreational activities.

The tools utilized by the specialist may differ slightly from those used by your regular optometrist or ophthalmologist. Charts and lenses are employed to assess your level of visual function, determining the amount of usable vision and how effectively you can utilize it.

Subsequently, the specialist will introduce various visual aids, including both optical and non-optical options, and recommend techniques to optimize your vision. Optical aids encompass items such as magnifiers and digital technologies, while non-optical aids include objects with large print (such as phones and kitchen items) or improved task lighting. Visual techniques involve methods like eccentric fixation and scanning. (Covered in the next chapter.)

After identifying the optical and non-optical aids that best suit your needs, the specialist can refer you to an expert who will assist you in utilizing these aids effectively and implementing low vision techniques.

Rehabilitation Services

Rehabilitation services are designed to help individuals with vision loss identify and learn strategies that maximize the use of their remaining functional vision. Through structured training and the development of compensatory skills, individuals can adapt more effectively and maintain independence in daily life.

Occupational Therapists (OT) are licensed healthcare professionals who assist individuals in functioning more independently. Some OTs receive advanced training in low vision and specialize in teaching practical strategies for coping with vision impairment—such as using magnifiers, enhancing lighting, and

26

modifying the home or work environment. Their goal is to help individuals adapt to their surroundings and sustain their independence.

Vision Rehabilitation Therapists (VRT) specialize in teaching adaptive daily living skills, including reading with magnifiers, using assistive technology, organizing the home, and managing personal care and household tasks. They most commonly work through state and federal agencies that support individuals who are blind or visually impaired.

Areas of Rehabilitative Training

1. **Work**
   An occupational therapist can help modify the work environment and train individuals in the use of both optical and non-optical aids to support meaningful and purposeful employment.

2. **Home Management**
   Therapists provide training in adaptive independent living skills, which may include a home visit. They can assist with modifying lighting, rearranging furniture for safety and accessibility, and setting up visual aids. Kitchen adaptations might involve improved lighting, contrast enhancement, tactile markers, and large-print or high-visibility tools.

3. **Personal Care**
   Therapists can assist with organizing and labeling bathroom items and medications to ensure safe and accurate use. They may also recommend tools such as magnifying mirrors or electronic magnifiers to help with grooming, shaving, and make-up application.

4. **Communication**
   Individuals can benefit from accessible phones with large buttons or voice command features. Artificial intelligence (AI) devices—such as smart speakers—are especially useful in this area, offering voice-activated internet access, reminders, and information without the need for screen interaction.

5. **Community Access**
   Therapists can advise individuals with low vision on accessing transportation options and local services. This might include orientation strategies, paratransit eligibility, or using technology for navigation and scheduling.

Navigating the World with Orientation and Mobility Training

For those with more severe impairment, the guidance of an **Orientation and Mobility Specialist** becomes invaluable. Orientation and mobility training focus on fostering independence and safety, aiding individuals in navigating their homes and public spaces.

Assistive devices used for mobility may include electronic aids, canes, guide dogs, and other walking aids. These specialists teach visually impaired individuals to utilize their senses and any remaining vision, as well as the proper use of a cane.

Certified Orientation and Mobility Specialists provide strategies for indoor and outdoor movement. They assess homes and workplaces for safety and ease of movement, using this information to assist individuals in orienting themselves and moving successfully. This training extends to navigating urban areas like streets and public transportation.

The skills imparted by an Orientation and Mobility Specialist greatly enhance the confidence, independence, and safety of visually impaired individuals.

Supporting Mental Well-Being: Counseling Services

Psychiatric and social counseling services are not universally available at every low vision center. These supports typically fall under the roles of psychiatrists, psychologists, licensed counselors, and social workers. Individuals with visual impairments may struggle silently with emotional and psychological challenges that often go unrecognized by doctors, family members, or friends.

The emotional impact of vision loss is often intensified by additional health concerns, family dynamics, or difficult living situations. In such cases, professional counseling may be needed—beyond what rehabilitation therapists are trained to provide.

Research shows a clear link between the severity of vision loss and the likelihood of experiencing depression. The greater the impairment, the more likely an individual is to experience symptoms of sadness, isolation, or feeling of hopelessness.

Conversely, studies have also found that individuals who received low vision rehabilitation services reported fewer depressive symptoms. (1) This underscores the importance of connecting with supportive services early in the vision loss journey.

Several professionals may be involved in supporting your mental and emotional well-being:

- **Low Vision Counselors** provide emotional support and teach coping strategies to help individuals adjust to vision loss.
- **Social Workers or Case Managers** can help coordinate care, connect you to services, and assist with emotional, financial, or housing needs.

Above all, **remember to advocate for yourself**. Vision loss is not just a physical change—it can be a deeply emotional and personal experience. Seeking support is not a weakness; it's an important part of healing and adaptation.

Low Vision Services for Children: A Comprehensive Approach

Children and teenagers may experience low vision due to inherited conditions or those acquired early in life. These include pediatric cataracts, pediatric glaucoma, nystagmus, and inherited retinal dystrophies, like Stargardt's Disease. The nature and timing of the vision loss greatly influence the types of services needed.

The level and focus of low vision services will vary depending on the child's age at diagnosis. The concerns for an infant are very different from those of a school-aged child.

In the first year or two of life, the primary focus is on supporting **brain development and functional vision**. As children enter school, the emphasis shifts to literacy development, educational access, and adaptive skills for learning.

The importance of early diagnosis and intervention—both medical and rehabilitative—cannot be overstated. With timely support and consistent access to adaptive tools and services, children with low vision can thrive in school and beyond. Their futures can be just as rich, fulfilling, and productive as those of their sighted peers.

The Role of Teachers of the Visually Impaired

Rehabilitation therapists and **Teachers of the Visually Impaired (TVI)** who specialize in pediatric low vision bring essential expertise to this stage. They understand how children's visual systems develop and are trained to design therapies and learning strategies tailored to each child's unique needs.

Teachers of the visually impaired play an important role by integrating the diagnosis with information from other specialists and therapists, conducting their own functional assessments within the school setting. They become advocates for the students, interpreting medical information and comprehending the unique needs of each low vision student. This information is then communicated to the educational team, ensuring that the student has appropriate access to academic learning.

These specialists collaborate closely with the student, family, and members of the child's educational team—including classroom teachers, orientation and mobility specialists, and school psychologists. Together, they create an **individualized educational plan (IEP)** or **Section 504 plan** that ensures the child receives appropriate instruction, accommodations, and support.

▤ **Note to Parents**: If you're unsure about your child's legal rights to educational accommodations, refer to **Section 504 of the Rehabilitation Act** for guidance. (2)

When to Consider a Referral for Low Vision Services

A referral for low vision services is generally recommended when an individual's visual acuity falls below **20/40 (6/12)**, or when there is evidence of visual field loss or reduced contrast sensitivity, as determined during a comprehensive eye examination by an eye care professional.

However, numbers alone don't tell the whole story.

If vision loss is interfering with your daily activities, ability to work, or overall quality of life—even if your acuity is better than 20/40—it is appropriate to seek low vision services. Functional limitations matter just as much as clinical measurements.

In short: **if your vision is getting in the way of how you live, it's time to ask for help.**

In the End...

Specialists in low vision, rehabilitation, mobility, and counseling conduct thorough functional vision assessments. These evaluations explore how vision loss affects your daily activities, work, personal care, and psychological well-being.

Through this process, professionals can track your progress in developing visual compensatory skills and adaptations. The outcomes of these assessments form the basis for creating personalized low vision service plans.

These customized plans provide a clear roadmap for improving independence and enhancing quality of life. In fact, research conducted in a Veterans Affairs (VA) setting found that individuals who received both rehabilitation therapy and low vision devices had better outcomes than those who received devices alone. (3) This highlights the importance of a **comprehensive, team-based approach** to vision care.

If we did all the things we are

capable of doing, we would literally

astound ourselves. Thomas Edison

The following resources can help you locate eye care professionals, access low vision and rehabilitation services, explore financial assistance, and find support for internet accessibility and inclusive design.

Find an Eye Doctor

American Optometric Association (via BrightFocus Foundation)
Search for optometrists by ZIP code.   You searched for find optometrist | BrightFocus Foundation

American Academy of Ophthalmology — "The Eye MD Association"
Find board-certified ophthalmologists.
https://secure.aao.org/aao/find-ophthalmologist

WebMD — Physician Directory
Search for eye care specialists (optometrists and ophthalmologists) by name, specialty, or location.
http://doctor.webmd.com/

Resources: Getting Help for Vision Loss

Find a Low Vision Specialist

National Council of State Agencies for the Blind (NCSAB)
Use the NCSAB directory to find your state's department for low vision and rehabilitation services. Click on your state abbreviation to view contact

information.
http://www.ncsab.org/List/StateDirectors

Rehabilitation Services

Lions Clubs International

Lions Clubs are local, volunteer-run service organizations that offer support for vision, hearing, and health. Known as Helen Keller's "Knights of the Blind," Lions Clubs sponsor various programs, including Low Vision Centers that provide education and rehabilitation. Type into browser: **Find Lions Low Vison Center**, telephone number listed at the time of this writing: **866-319-9733**

Low Vision Services: APH Directory of Services Listings. This is a source for finding services in your state or province. In the dropdown select for Low Vision Services, then your state or province.
https://test.visionaware.org/directory/

Braille Institute: If you are in California, call to make an appointment with an occupational therapist: 866-866-8995

VA Blind Rehabilitation Services for eligible Veterans and active-duty Service members. Check their website. Low vision centers are not found in every state.

Financial Help

The following programs offer financial assistance for eye exams, eyeglasses, and access to essential vision care services, particularly for those who are uninsured, underinsured, or low-income.

USA.gov **SSDI and SSI benefits for people with disabilities**

https://www.usa.gov/social-security-disability

Social Security Administration (SSA) Provides information on Social Security Disability Insurance (SSDI) and Supplemental Security Income (SSI). Includes a Benefits Eligibility Tool and instructions for applying online or by phone.

www.ssa.gov/disability

EyeCare America
A public service program of the American Academy of Ophthalmology offering free eye exams through volunteer ophthalmologists. Use the online eligibility questionnaire to determine if you qualify.
www.eyecareamerica.org

New Eyes for the Needy
Offers free eyeglasses to individuals in financial need. Applicants must have a current eyeglass prescription. A voucher request must be submitted by a social service agency, school nurse, or similar professional.
www.new-eyes.org
New Eyes Glasses (for redeeming vouchers)

OneSight – OnSight Voucher Program
An independent nonprofit offering free eyeglasses through participating Luxottica retail locations (e.g., LensCrafters, Target Optical, Pearle Vision). Requirements:

- Must be referred by a verified 501(c)(3) nonprofit (e.g., Lions Club, Red Cross, school, church)
- Referral letter must be on organization letterhead and include a Tax ID number
- Valid prescription (less than 2 years old) required
  If an exam is needed, patients may request a donated exam from the retailer's on-site doctor or contact Prevent Blindness for help.

https://rma.pointcomfort.com/files/OneSight%20Voucher%20Program%20Intro.pdf?utm_source=chatgpt.com or type into your browser: OneSight Voucher Program

Internet Accessibility for the Visually Impaired and Website Designers

Online access is essential for education, work, and daily life. These resources support individuals with vision loss and help website designers understand how to create accessible digital content.

MyVision.org — Improve Internet Accessibility
Offers guidance on making websites more accessible to people with impaired vision, including practical design tips and accessibility standards.
https://myvision.org/guides/internet-accessibility-guide/

For Students with Disabilities

Intelligent.com — College Planning Guide for Students with Learning Disabilities
This comprehensive guide covers college preparation, financial aid, accommodations, and advocacy tips for students with disabilities, including those with visual impairments.
www.intelligent.com/college-planning-guide-for-students-with-learning-disabilities

References

1. Rovner BW, Casten RJ, Hegel MT, Massof RW, Leiby BE, Ho AC, Tasman WS. Low vision depression prevention trial in age-related macular degeneration: a randomized clinical trial. Ophthalmology. 2014 Nov;121(11):2204-11. doi: 10.1016/j.ophtha.2014.05.002. Epub 2014 Jul 9. PMID: 25016366; PMCID: PMC4253064

2. U.S. Department of Education. Section 504. Home > Laws and Policies > Individuals with Disabilities

3. Stelmack JA, Tang XC, Wei Y, Wilcox DT, Morand T, Brahm K, Sayers S, Massof RW; LOVIT II Study Group. Outcomes of the Veterans Affairs Low Vision Intervention Trial II (LOVIT II): A Randomized Clinical Trial. JAMA Ophthalmol. 2017 Feb 1;135(2):96-104. doi: 10.1001/jamaophthalmol.2016.4742. PMID: 27978569.

Low Vision Training: Relearning How to See

Low vision therapy exercises are specialized training exercises crafted to assist visually impaired individuals in utilizing their remaining vision effectively, with or without devices. These exercises aim to optimize the use of residual vision, improving the ability to carry out activities of daily living (ADL).

These exercises are typically conducted under the guidance of a vision rehabilitation specialist or an occupational therapist, tailored to the individual's specific needs and the nature of their visual impairment.

Several factors can influence the success of vision training. Age, motivation, family support, depression, and living circumstances can either facilitate or hinder the learning process.

It's important to note that progress in vision training is *gradual*. Learning new skills may require 2 to 4 weeks of daily practice. During this time, the visually impaired individual may experience feelings of frustration, discouragement, or impatience. Those with more severe vision loss may require an extended period to learn how to best utilize their residual vision.

Training the Eyes and Mind: Essential Low Vision Techniques

Vision loss affects people in many different ways—ranging from central vision loss, peripheral vision loss, blurry vision, or difficulty with contrast and light sensitivity. Because of this diversity, vision therapy exercises must be personalized to match each individual's visual challenges and daily goals.

While glasses or contact lenses may help with refractive errors, most types of low vision—such as that caused by macular degeneration, diabetic retinopathy, glaucoma, and inherited retinal diseases—cannot be fully corrected. Instead, the focus shifts to enhancing the use of remaining vision. This is where low vision rehabilitation exercises can play a key role.

1. Learning to Use Low Vision Tools Effectively

Low vision devices include a wide range of tools, from simple hand-held magnifiers to advanced video magnifiers, computer-based software, wearable telescopes, and electronic glasses. These tools can be life-changing, but proper training is essential to use them effectively and avoid frustration.

Training typically covers the following:

- **Eyewear compatibility** – Should the device be used with your prescription glasses?
- **Intended use** – Is the device designed for near tasks (like reading) or distance viewing?
- **Working distance** – How far from your eyes should the device be held?
- **Device handling** – How to position and stabilize the device for best results.
- **Lighting optimization** – What type of lighting works best, and where should it be placed?
- **Advanced features** – How to use optional settings such as contrast modes, zoom, or text-to-speech functions.

Training often involves some trial and error, especially when devices are purchased online without professional guidance. If you or someone you care for is struggling with a device, it may not be the right match—or it simply might not be used correctly. Professional instruction can make a significant difference in success and satisfaction.

2. Eccentric Viewing Training Exercises

Eccentric viewing training is especially helpful for individuals with central vision loss caused by conditions such as macular degeneration, diabetic retinopathy, or inherited retinal diseases.

These exercises teach individuals how to make use of the healthier peripheral areas of the retina—parts of the visual field that are not damaged by disease. Although peripheral vision does not offer the same level of detail or clarity as central vision, it can still be highly functional, particularly when combined with magnification devices.

With practice, a person can learn to shift their gaze slightly to one side of the target object so that the image falls on a functioning part of the retina. This area is referred to as the **preferred retinal locus (PRL)**. Eccentric viewing exercises help individuals identify this "new" seeing spot and train their eyes and brain to use it more efficiently for everyday tasks such as reading, facial recognition, or watching TV.

Location of eccentric viewing areas:

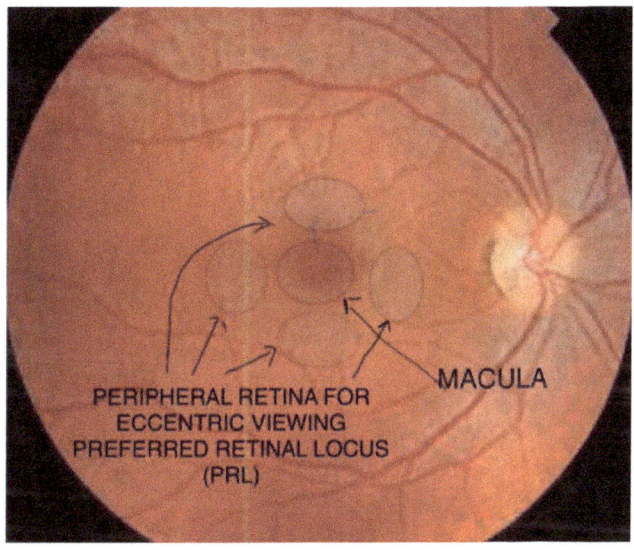

PERIPHERAL RETINA FOR
ECCENTRIC VIEWING
PREFERRED RETINAL LOCUS
(PRL)

MACULA

Mastering eccentric viewing enables individuals to better utilize magnifying devices and enhances their ability to navigate their environment independently.

Interestingly, I've observed that younger individuals with visual impairments and those who experience a gradual loss of vision often naturally develop eccentric viewing skills without formal instruction or training. For others, targeted training from a low vision therapist can greatly accelerate progress and improve confidence in daily life.

3. Training Orientation and Mobility

Orientation and mobility (O&M) training teaches individuals how to understand their position in space (**orientation**) and move safely and efficiently through their environment (**mobility**). These essential life skills are taught by certified Orientation and Mobility Specialists.

This training is particularly beneficial for individuals who are blind or who have severely restricted peripheral vision, such as those with retinitis pigmentosa, end-stage glaucoma, or advanced diabetic retinopathy.

O&M Training Techniques:

1. The Sighted Guide Technique

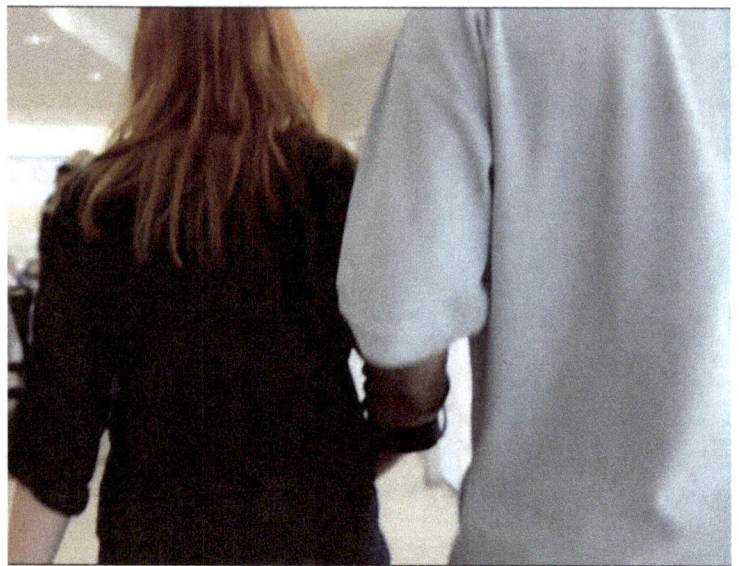

In this method, the individual with low vision grasps the arm of a trained guide just above the elbow, walking slightly behind and to the side of the guide. The guide provides verbal cues or uses arm movements to signal upcoming obstacles, such as door frames, stairs, curbs, and narrow passages.

Vision Awareness Training YouTube Video

2. The Long (White) Cane

The long cane is a symbol of independence. The user sweeps it in a rhythmic arc to detect changes in terrain and avoid obstacles. It enables people with visual impairment to move independently and safely.

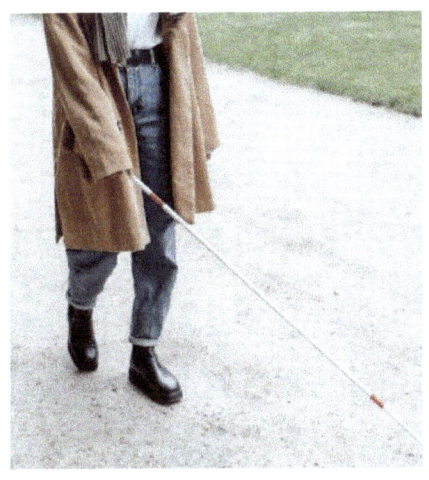

The white cane also serves as a public identifier of visual disability. In the United States, **white cane laws** vary by state, but typically grant users the legal "right of way." It's important that both cane users and drivers understand the relevant laws in their state regarding when to stop, yield, or proceed with caution.

Smart canes, which incorporate electronic sensors, provide additional features such as detecting obstacles above waist level and offering feedback through vibrations (haptics) or audio navigation.

3. Guide Dogs

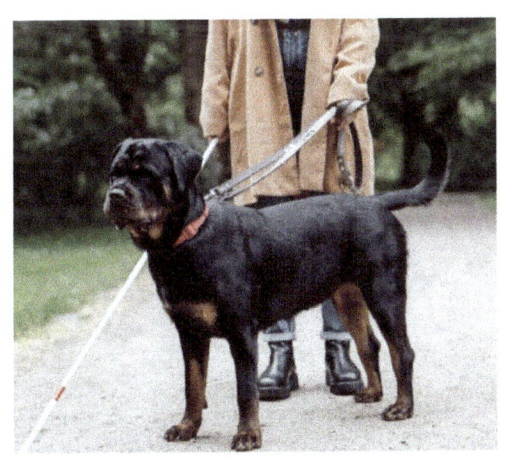

Guide dogs are specially trained animals that assist individuals with severe vision loss. Dogs are carefully screened for temperament, focus, and trainability. Once selected, they undergo rigorous training before being matched with a handler.

To qualify for a guide dog, individuals must already possess strong orientation and mobility skills. They must also be prepared to learn dog-handling techniques and commit to maintaining the dog's training and well-being.

4. Electronic Navigation Devices

Modern O&M training often includes instruction in the use of electronic navigation tools. Devices like the **Victor Reader Trek** or smartphone apps with GPS and step-by-step navigation can significantly enhance independence.

While powerful, these devices do have a learning curve. O&M specialists can help users integrate technology into daily life safely and effectively.

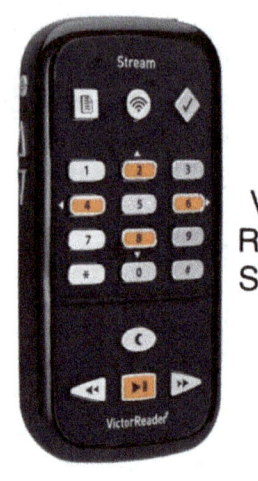

Victor
Reader
Stream

Victor Reader Trekker

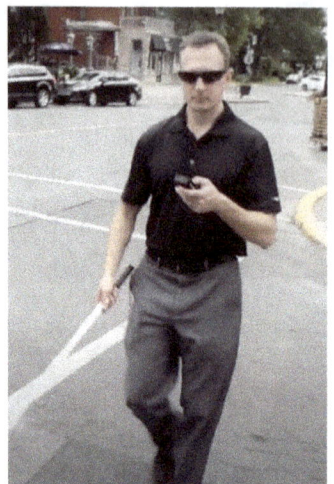

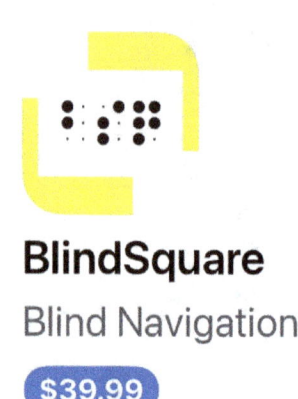

BlindSquare

Blind Navigation

$39.99

Blindsquare for smartphone

4. Tracking and Scanning Exercises for Low Vision

These exercises help individuals develop better eye movement control and improve the use of residual vision.

Tracking moving objects with the eyes helps to improve eye movement coordination and tracking abilities. This can help with reading skills and using low vision devices proficiently.

Scanning skills help with the localization of objects both near and at a distance. Someone with low vision can become more efficient and more independent using eye movement to scan their environment. This is especially helpful for those who have lost much of their peripheral vision.

Together, these skills contribute to more efficient navigation and greater visual independence.

5. Training in the Use of Bioptic Telescopes for Driving

Driving with low vision is a complex and highly regulated issue. In the United States, each state sets its own laws governing whether individuals with visual impairments may drive using assistive devices such as **bioptic telescopes**. While this practice is permitted in some states, it remains controversial and is strictly prohibited in others.

Bioptic telescopes are small, high-powered lenses mounted onto glasses that allow users to spot distant objects—such as road signs or traffic signals—by briefly glancing through the telescope, while using their regular lenses for general navigation.

In states where **bioptic driving is legal**, individuals must first undergo a comprehensive evaluation by a low vision specialist or vision rehabilitation professional. This assessment determines whether the person meets the visual and cognitive criteria for bioptic driving.

If approved, the individual begins specialized training with a certified driving instructor. This training includes:

- Learning how to safely alternate between the carrier lens and telescope.
- Developing the timing and judgment needed to use the telescope briefly and appropriately/.
- Practicing real-world driving scenarios under supervision.
- Meeting all state-specific vision and driving requirements.

Bioptic driving training is rigorous and individualized. It demands a high level of visual awareness, coordination, and safety consciousness, and it may not be suitable for everyone. However, for some individuals, it represents a life-changing opportunity to regain independence.

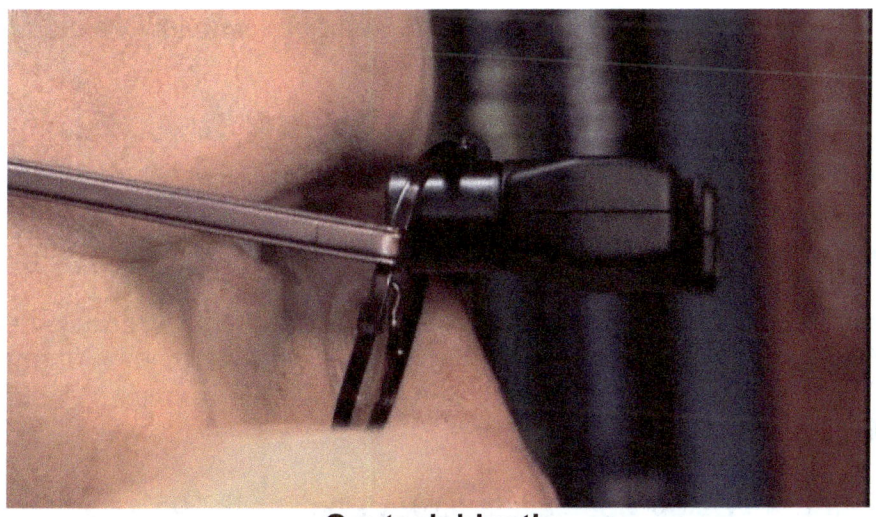

Ocutech bioptic

Who Needs Low Vision Training—and Why?

Low vision training can be immensely beneficial for individuals living with conditions such as macular degeneration, diabetic retinopathy, retinitis pigmentosa, glaucoma, and other vision-related disorders. People with these conditions often face daily challenges with reading, recognizing faces, moving through unfamiliar spaces, and maintaining their independence.

By learning to use visual aids, adaptive technology, and compensatory techniques, individuals can regain confidence, improve their safety, and enhance their quality of life.

Low vision training is not limited to those with long-standing vision loss. It can also be valuable for individuals experiencing *gradual* changes in vision. As eyesight declines, learning new strategies early can ease the transition and help preserve independence for as long as possible.

Where can someone with low vision get low vision training?

Individuals with low vision can receive low vision training from various sources and often involves a team of professionals who specialize in vision rehabilitation. Here are some places where someone with low vision can access training:

1. **Rehabilitation Centers:** Many countries have rehabilitation centers or clinics that specialize in vision rehabilitation. These centers often have a team of professionals, including orientation and mobility specialists, occupational therapists, and low vision therapists, who can provide training and support.

2. **Specialized Schools for the Blind or Visually Impaired:** Some regions have schools specifically designed for individuals with visual impairments. These schools may offer comprehensive vision rehabilitation services, including low vision training.

3. **Private Low Vision Specialists:** Low vision specialists, often optometrists or ophthalmologists, may provide individualized low vision assessments and training. These professionals can prescribe and teach how to use low vision aids and devices.

4. **Local Rehabilitation Services:** In many areas, local government or nonprofit organizations provide rehabilitation services for the disabled, including those with low vision. These services may include training in daily living skills, mobility training, and how to use assistive technology.

5. **Occupational Therapists:** Occupational therapists, who specialize in low vision rehabilitation, can provide training to help individuals adapt and develop strategies for daily activities.

6. **Support Groups and Non-profit Organizations:** Joining local or online support groups for individuals with visual impairments can be a valuable resource. Some nonprofit organizations, like the Lion's Club, are dedicated to supporting the visually impaired may offer training programs or connect individuals with appropriate services.

Additionally, local government agencies and organizations for the visually impaired may have information on available resources in the community.

Tip: Local government agencies, disability services offices, and organizations for the visually impaired often maintain directories of available low vision resources in the community. These are good starting points for anyone seeking training or referrals.

In The End...

Low vision therapy exercises are a vital part of vision rehabilitation. These techniques empower individuals to make the most of their remaining vision while learning adaptive strategies for everyday life. The ultimate goal is to improve functional ability and enhance quality of life.

By acquiring these skills, people with low vision can maintain independence, preserve self-sufficiency, and support their emotional and social well-being. With the right training and support, individuals can continue to live full and meaningful lives—even in the face of significant vision loss.

The Experience of Vision Loss

Adjusting to Vision Loss, 7 Keys to Coping

Adjusting to vision loss is a deeply personal and transformative journey. It involves shifting your focus from what has been lost to what remains possible. This process is not about denial—it's about discovering new ways to live fully and meaningfully.

Coping with vision loss involves more than just practical changes; it requires emotional and psychological adjustment. The seven keys to this adjustment include managing stress, maintaining a positive attitude, building strong social connections, keeping the mind engaged, continuing to learn, seeking professional support, and embracing humor along the way.

While the road can be difficult, recognizing what you *can* change—and accepting what you can't—is a powerful first step toward regaining control and confidence in your life.

1. Reduce Stress

Adjusting to vision loss can be emotionally and practically overwhelming. The uncertainty, new challenges, and changes in independence can create significant stress. However, adopting proactive strategies can help you manage this stress and build resilience during your transition. Below are effective ways to reduce stress while adapting to vision loss:

- **Organize Your Environment**
  Simplify your living space by arranging items in a consistent, logical way. Label drawers, use tactile markers, and keep frequently used items in predictable places. A well-organized environment minimizes frustration and supports daily function.
- **Use Assistive Technology**
  Embrace tools that promote independence—such as screen readers, magnifiers, and voice-controlled devices. These technologies can ease the stress caused by inaccessibility and help you regain control over daily activities.

- **Practice Mindfulness and Relaxation**
  Techniques like meditation, deep breathing, or guided imagery can help reduce anxiety and create a sense of calm. Regular mindfulness practice supports emotional balance through difficult moments.
- **Seek Emotional Support**
  Talk to friends, family, or connect with support groups—especially those focused on vision loss. Sharing your experiences with others who understand can provide comfort, validation, and encouragement.
- **Set Realistic Goals**
  Break tasks into manageable steps and celebrate small successes. Focusing on progress, rather than perfection, can reduce stress and build confidence.
- **Maintain a Healthy Lifestyle**
  Physical health strongly influences emotional well-being. Regular exercise, nutritious meals, and adequate sleep can help you manage stress more effectively.
- **Engage in Enjoyable Activities**
  Make time for hobbies or pastimes that bring joy and fulfillment—like listening to music, creating art, gardening, or spending time in nature. Enjoyable activities offer mental relief and a renewed sense of purpose.
- **Practice Self-Compassion**
  Be gentle with yourself as you adjust. It's normal to experience a range of emotions. Recognize your effort and strength—it takes courage to adapt to a new reality.
- **Plan Ahead and Stay Organized**
  Establish routines and use planning tools like calendars or reminders to keep daily life on track. Anticipating and preparing for tasks and appointments reduces last-minute stress and promotes a sense of control.

Reducing stress lays a strong foundation for coping with vision loss—but stress management alone is not enough. How you *think* about your situation can profoundly shape how you *feel* and *adapt*. That's why the next key to adjusting is developing a positive, resilient attitude.

2. Adopting a Resilient Outlook

Your mindset plays an important role in how you cope with vision loss. Emotional reactions vary widely, and people respond to this life change in many different ways. Understanding these different responses—and recognizing where you fall along the spectrum—can help you move toward **acceptance** and growth.

Below are common mindsets people may experience when dealing with vision loss:

- **The Deniers**
  Deniers avoid facing the reality of their vision loss. They may blame others or external circumstances, refuse to acknowledge the changes they're experiencing, or resist using low vision devices and assistive tools. They often keep their vision loss a secret and cling to hope for a quick fix or cure. This denial may prevent them from taking important steps toward adaptation and can lead to ongoing frustration and emotional distress. For these individuals, professional support can be an essential first step toward acceptance.

- **The Angry**
  Anger is a natural reaction to losing vision—but some people get stuck in it. They may feel that life has become unfair or that they've lost control. Unfortunately, remaining in a state of bitterness or resentment doesn't change the reality. The key is learning to redirect that anger into action—whether by seeking help, advocating for your needs, or learning new skills to regain independence.

- **The Helpless**
  Those who feel helpless may struggle with low self-worth and become dependent on others, often withdrawing from responsibilities and daily challenges. Sometimes, they receive unintended reinforcement through extra attention or support, which may keep them from moving forward. With encouragement—and possibly guidance from vision rehabilitation specialists or counselors—they can begin to reclaim independence in their lives.

- **The Resigned**
  Individuals in this category have accepted that their vision has changed, but they've stopped there. They may feel that life will never be the same, and that there's little point in trying. They often experience ongoing grief or depression and avoid activities that now seem too difficult. But acceptance without action is only half the journey. These individuals are on the path—but with the right tools and encouragement, they can still find meaning, purpose, and joy.

- **The Adapters**
  Finally, there are those that see their impairment as a challenge, and as something they just have to deal with. They have **accepted** it, they are **adjusting**, and are **adapting**. Life goes on. "Everybody's got somethin'." What doesn't kill me makes me stronger." These individuals have a

willingness to accept the help of low vision professionals and accessibility devices.

It's common to cycle through many of these attitudes as you adjust to vision loss. Some days may be harder than others, and that's okay. The important thing is to recognize where you are emotionally—and to set a goal to keep moving forward: to **accept**, **adjust**, and **adapt**.

3. You Are Not Alone: The Importance of Staying Connected

While adopting a resilient outlook is essential, it doesn't mean going it alone. Vision loss often carries emotional weight—fears about the future, the burden of stigma, the loss of independence—and can easily lead to isolation. The less you interact with others, the more inward you may turn. Feelings of sadness, low self-esteem, and loneliness can grow stronger when left unspoken.

But you are not alone.

Even if you have a supportive family, connecting with others who are also experiencing vision loss—or other disabilities—can be uniquely helpful. Family and friends may listen and try to understand your fears and concerns and try to help where they can. But, be aware that there may be an expiration date on their capability to listen to complaints, rants, whining, and demands on their time That doesn't mean they don't love you—it just means you may need a broader circle of support.

Talking to others with similar experiences can help you process your emotions and feel seen. That's exactly why support groups exist. They provide a safe space to share your concerns, listen to others' stories, and realize that your fears and frustrations are not unique or shameful. Knowing others face similar struggles can be comforting and empowering.

If traditional support groups don't appeal to you, consider connecting with individuals who have other types of disabilities. Many people with visual impairment don't know anyone else with the same condition—but disability, in general, creates shared psychological and social challenges. You may find deep understanding and camaraderie in surprising places, even among people with very different life stories. Swapping "war stories" can be cathartic and help reveal both your strengths and areas where you may still need support.

If your circumstances limit access to in-person interaction, the internet offers meaningful alternatives. Online forums, blogs, and message boards focused on low vision and specific eye conditions provide spaces to read, share, and learn. Sometimes just knowing someone else shares your challenges can bring a powerful sense of connection.

4. Engage Your Mind with Purpose

Do you ever wake up, move through the house aimlessly, and realize the day is passing without meaning or momentum? Maybe you turn on the TV and think, "I'm doing something... I'm watching or listening." And that's okay—for a while.

But eventually, passively passing time isn't enough.

Self-help experts and psychologists agree: to feel self-worth, we need a sense of purpose. Purpose doesn't have to mean a career or major project—it can be found in setting goals, pursuing hobbies, learning something new, creating, volunteering, or simply taking on daily responsibilities. Try engaging your brain with puzzles, audiobooks, or creative tasks like writing or crafting.

These small efforts help fight off despair and restore a sense of control.

Your vision loss won't disappear. It will show up throughout the day to remind you of its presence. But how you respond to those reminders is what shapes your ability to cope and thrive.

Engaging your mind gives you more than just distraction—it gives you direction. And one of the most empowering ways to stay mentally active is through learning. Knowledge doesn't just inform—it equips you to make better choices, advocate for yourself, and feel more in control of your future.

5. Knowledge is Empowering

Knowledge truly is power. The more you learn, the more equipped you are to make informed decisions, face challenges, and take control of your life. I once had a college professor tell me, "You can argue any point with me—if you've done your homework." That advice stuck with me.

You don't have to become an expert in low vision or the medical details of your condition. But you *can* learn enough to understand how your vision loss affects you—and how to work around it. The more you understand your disability, the better prepared you are to adapt, advocate, and find solutions.

Today, information is more accessible than ever. Assistive technologies are increasingly sophisticated and user-friendly. And while public awareness still has room to grow, it's improving—and with it, opportunities are expanding for people with disabilities.

The more you know, the more capable and confident you can become.

6. Seek Professional Guidance

No one has all the answers—and you shouldn't be expected to go it alone. Fortunately, a wide range of professionals specialize in different aspects of disability and vision loss. Each brings unique expertise to help you navigate the emotional, physical, and practical challenges of adapting to vision changes.

As you reorganize your life and face evolving psychological and social issues, your needs may shift. Having access to the right professionals at the right time can make a significant difference.

A great starting point is a low vision specialist or rehabilitation team. These professionals are not only experts in vision care—they also understand how to connect you with state agencies, community resources, support groups, and organizations dedicated to helping individuals with disabilities. Often, the biggest barrier is simply knowing these services exist.

The most powerful advocate for your needs is *you*. When you're **informed, supported, and connected** to the right professionals, you're better equipped to build the life you want.

While professional guidance provides essential tools and support, maintaining your emotional well-being requires more than expertise—it calls for resilience, optimism, and sometimes, a little laughter.

54

7. Maintain a Sense of Humor

Years ago, I heard a woman on a self-help CD say she helped herself through cancer by watching funny movies and making sure she laughed every day. I can't say laughter cured her illness, but I do believe it's good medicine for the soul.

When facing the challenges that come with vision loss, it's easy to get overwhelmed by negative emotions. Lifting yourself up can be difficult, but maintaining a sense of humor doesn't mean you need to become a comedian. It's more about cultivating a mindset that allows you to set aside negative thoughts, even temporarily, and find lightness in life's situations.

This might mean seeking out stress-relieving activities, enjoying positive friendships, spending time with loving pets, or simply appreciating entertainment that makes you smile. Whatever it is that brings you joy and laughter, make room for it in your life.

A sense of humor can be a powerful source of strength—helping you cope, connect, and keep moving forward.

In the End...

As you navigate the journey of adjusting to vision loss, remember this: your disability does not define you. It is only one part of who you are—not the whole story. You remain a person fully capable of enjoying life's pleasures and sharing in laughter.

Start by learning to not take yourself too seriously and by welcoming positive thoughts into your daily life. Your vision loss does not diminish your worth or the richness of the experiences still ahead. So, as you move forward embrace your whole self—disabilities--and all and continue to live a life filled with joy, laughter, and resilience.

> *"Ask and it will be given to you;*
> *seek and you will find;*
> *knock and the door will be opened to you."*
> Mattheo 7:7-8 New King James Bible

How Vision Loss Affects the Social, Emotional, and Practical Aspects of Life

Vision loss has profound effects on various aspects of life, influencing independence, self-perception, relationships, communication, economic status, expectations, and goals. Tasks that were once effortless now become challenging and time-consuming.

Navigating Independence with Vision Loss

Loss of independence due to vision loss can manifest in two primary forms: an inability to perform daily tasks without assistance and a decline in freedom of mobility.

In our daily lives, the human eye effortlessly guides us through routine tasks with minimal forethought. Tasks such as personal care, medication management, reading, and household chores fall under the umbrella of activities of daily living. However, for those experiencing vision loss, these tasks must be approached differently, potentially leading to dependence on others for completion.

Fortunately, independence can often be preserved through training and a willingness to adapt by utilizing visual aids or adjusting living environments to suit individual needs.

Initially, acknowledging the need for assistance can be challenging, especially for individuals accustomed to a life with sight. While adjustments can be made to the living environment, there will inevitably be moments when external help is necessary. In these instances, it's important to accept assistance to make challenging tasks more manageable.

Sometimes, well-intentioned family and friends may feel compelled to offer excessive help, inadvertently taking over tasks that the visually impaired person is capable of handling themselves. This can lead to a sense of helplessness and loss of control, ultimately *increasing* dependency.

It's important to resist the temptation to allow others to take over tasks that can still be managed independently. Maintaining even a semblance of independence is pivotal in retaining control over various aspects of life.

For those whose visual acuity falls below 20/40—the legal limit for driving—one of the most profound losses is the ability to drive. Suddenly, the freedom to come and go at will is gone. Individuals must rely on others for transportation to run errands, attend appointments, or participate in daily activities—an adjustment that can feel frustrating and disempowering. In areas without accessible public transit, this dependency often leads to social isolation, which in turn can trigger a cascade of negative emotions.

In cases of profound vision loss, individuals may also face significant challenges with **orientation and mobility**. *Orientation* refers to understanding one's position within the environment, while *mobility* involves the ability to move safely and independently through that space. Without clear visual cues, navigating even familiar areas can become daunting. Fear of getting lost, disoriented, or stranded is common and can further discourage people from venturing out.

To manage these difficulties, many people with severe visual impairments rely on tools such as white canes or guide dogs to maintain as much independence as possible. These aids not only help with navigation but also provide a sense of security and confidence in unfamiliar or crowded environments.

How Vision Impairment Affects Self-perception

Losing vision after having once been sighted can be an overwhelming experience, often bringing a wave of negative emotions. Whether they were a skilled worker, a parent, or socially active, the sudden loss of vision can leave them feeling overwhelmed and concerned about their quality of life and financial stability.

Self-perception is strongly influenced by how others react to and treat them. When co-workers, family, and friends begin to treat them differently, it can lead to feelings of stigmatization, reinforcing a sense of being defined by their disability.

A decline in self-esteem and confidence is common. Independence may give way to dependence, and the loss of control over daily life can create feelings of diminished worth. Many begin to doubt their abilities as workers, parents, or partners, questioning their value and capability.

However, as individuals adapt to their new reality, their self-perception often shifts. Learning new skills and finding ways to navigate their environment can ease the burden of vision loss. Gaining independence through these adaptations not only enhances their ability to function in daily life but also rebuilds self-confidence and fosters a renewed sense of purpose.

How Vision Loss Affects Relationships

Relationships with family and friends are important for individuals who are visually impaired. Their understanding, acceptance, and willingness to assist play a pivotal role in the adjustment process for those with visual disabilities.

Navigating life without support can be significantly more challenging for visually impaired individuals compared to those with a supportive family environment. Friends and responsive healthcare providers can also offer the encouragement and support necessary for the individual to regain independence.

However, support from family and friends is not always guaranteed. When a loved one loses their vision, family members may struggle to accept the changes in roles and routines that follow. The dynamics within the household inevitably shift. Tasks that were once shared—such as cooking, cleaning, running errands, or driving—may now fall primarily on one or two individuals who assume a caregiving role. These changes can also introduce financial strain, as responsibilities increase and income sources may be affected.

Complicating matters, the visually impaired person may still appear "normal" to others and manage many tasks independently. As a result, some family members may underestimate the extent of the impairment or even deny that a problem exists. This lack of understanding can discourage the individual from asking for help, especially if their family's expectations have not adapted to their new reality. The emotional toll of this disconnect can be profound, particularly for someone already coping with anxiety or depression.

On the other hand, some family members may swing to the opposite extreme—feeling compelled to take over and manage even the simplest tasks for the visually impaired individual. They may hover and assist with every step, often with good intentions, but this can inadvertently undermine the person's independence and contribute to feelings of incompetence. Over time, such dynamics can erode self-esteem and foster resentment or helplessness.

Social situations bring their own set of challenges. Friends and extended family may not fully understand what low vision entails, leading to frequent misunderstandings. A visually impaired person may struggle to recognize faces or see details clearly, which can cause others to wrongly perceive them as aloof, clumsy, or even unintelligent. In public settings, such as stores or restaurants, clerks and staff may grow impatient with delayed responses or hesitant movements, further adding to feelings of inadequacy.

When these incidents occur repeatedly, they can chip away at the individual's social confidence. Over time, this can lead to withdrawal from social activities, increasing the risk of isolation, depression, and anxiety—a cycle that is often hard to break without external support.

Supporting Healthier Family Dynamics

Improving family communication is essential for navigating the emotional and practical challenges that come with vision loss. Open, respectful dialogue helps reduce misunderstandings and prevents resentment from building. Visually impaired individuals should feel empowered to express their needs, limitations, and preferences honestly—while family members, in turn, must be willing to listen without judgment or assumption. Family meetings or informal check-ins can create a safe space for sharing frustrations, adjusting expectations, and solving problems together.

Education also plays a key role. When family members learn more about low vision—what it means functionally and emotionally—they're better equipped to offer meaningful, balanced support. Resources from organizations such as the **American Foundation for the Blind (AFB)**, **National Federation of the Blind (NFB)**, and **VisionAware** can provide helpful insights, reading materials, and workshops.

For some families, seeking guidance from a counselor, social worker, or vision rehabilitation therapist can be transformative. These professionals can help mediate difficult conversations, teach adaptive strategies, and assist the family in setting realistic, shared goals. Low vision clinics often have mental health professionals or support services integrated into their care teams.

Finally, support groups—both in-person and online—can offer a valuable outlet for visually impaired individuals and their family members. Sharing experiences with others who are going through similar challenges can reduce feelings of isolation and foster a sense of community. Many people find emotional relief and practical solutions through these connections.

How Low Vision Affects Communication

Individuals with low vision—especially those with central vision loss—are often categorized as **"print disabled."** It's easy to underestimate just how much of daily life depends on access to printed information. From work documents and personal correspondence to labels, signs, and instructions, print is everywhere.

Think about the countless places printed information appears: TV screens, product packaging, street signs, and even the numbers on appliance dials. For someone with a print disability, each of these can become a barrier to communication and independence. (And yes, this category also includes individuals with **dyslexia**.)

While magnification often offers a partial solution, it's important to recognize that there is no universal tool that works for every situation. The challenge—for the visually impaired, their caregivers, and low vision specialists—is to find the most effective combination of aids, including magnifiers, audio devices, and environmental adaptations. These tools are essential for gathering information and navigating the world with confidence.

Fortunately, today's generation of visually impaired individuals has access to powerful assistive technology. Modern smartphones, tablets, and computers come equipped with accessibility features designed to support those with visual, hearing, and mobility impairments. However, simply having access to these tools isn't enough—proper setup, customization, and training are crucial to using them effectively.

Even with these advancements, one of the most difficult communication challenges remains: recognizing faces. Central vision loss often impairs facial recognition, which can lead to uncomfortable or even embarrassing social encounters. Human communication relies not just on words and tone, but also on subtle visual cues—like facial expressions—that convey emotion and intent. When these non-verbal cues are missed, interactions can feel strained or incomplete. Sadly, no assistive technology currently offers a fully effective solution for this aspect of communication.

How Vision Loss Changes Expectations and Goals

There's a saying: "We make plans, and God just laughs." It captures the uncertainty of life—and the way vision loss can unexpectedly alter the path we imagined for ourselves. As humans, we're wired to look forward. Each day, we're driven by plans and goals, whether they involve family and home life, career aspirations, or leisure activities like travel or sports.

Parents of children with low vision, like all parents, have hopes for their child's growth, education, and independence. But when vision loss enters the picture, some of these expectations may need to shift. For many, especially those who experience sudden or traumatic vision loss, this adjustment brings understandable grief, sadness, or even fear for the future. In contrast, those with gradual or progressive vision loss may have more time to emotionally prepare and reframe their goals over time.

Support from counselors, therapists, or vision rehabilitation specialists can be invaluable during this period of adjustment. These professionals can help individuals develop new strategies for achieving personal, academic, work-related, and recreational goals—goals that reflect both their evolving abilities and their enduring strengths.

As this process unfolds, individuals often learn to let go of outdated expectations and embrace new possibilities. Focusing on what *can* be done—rather than what's been lost—can be profoundly empowering. Channeling energy into meaningful, enjoyable activities fosters both skill development and emotional resilience.

Parents naturally worry about their child's future. Fortunately, in the United States, federal legislation such as **Section 504** of the **Rehabilitation Act** of 1973 guarantees educational access and accommodations for children with disabilities. Additional state and federal programs provide support for eligible students through age 21. (See Reference 1: "Parents' Information and Resources" for a state-by-state listing.)

The Financial Impact of Vision Loss

The costs associated with vision impairment can be significant. Loss of employment due to declining vision can have a devastating financial impact—not only on the individual, but on their entire family. In addition to lost income, the added costs of medical care, assistive devices, and, in some cases, personal caregivers, can place further strain on household finances.

Fortunately, there are government and state programs that offer financial assistance, particularly for educational and rehabilitation services. Medical care is typically covered by health insurance—whether through private providers or public programs like Medicaid and Medicare. However, it's important to note that **eyeglasses, low vision aids, and assistive technology are often not covered**, leaving these expenses to be paid out of pocket. For a list of helpful financial resources, see the chapter' *Where to Get Help When You Have Vision Loss* final section—Resources, which includes sources for a state-by-state directory of available services.

In some cases, vision impairment does not mean giving up a career. With the right accommodations and tools, many individuals with low vision or blindness are able to continue working successfully, depending on their field and the severity of their vision loss. Advancements in technology—such as screen readers, magnification software, and adaptive workstations—have made it more possible than ever to remain employed.

The Americans with Disabilities Act (ADA) provides protection in the workplace. Under ADA guidelines, employers with 15 or more employees are required to make *reasonable accommodations* for workers with vision disabilities, as long as the employee can still perform the essential functions of the job safely and effectively. For more information, see the U.S. Equal Employment Opportunity Commission's *Fact Sheet: Disability Discrimination* (Reference 2).

How to Maintain Quality of Life

Vision loss is one of the most feared disabilities, and understandably so—it can affect nearly every aspect of a person's life. Independence, self-image, relationships, communication, and financial stability can all be disrupted in ways that are deeply personal and difficult to anticipate.

If these challenges are left unaddressed, they can lead to a cascade of emotional distress. Feelings of fear, anxiety, depression, loneliness, and helplessness are common after vision loss, and they can significantly hinder the process of acceptance, adjustment, and adaptation.

However, many individuals do learn to cope and even thrive. Those who tend to fare best often share certain traits: a strong sense of **self-worth, emotional flexibility, and a willingness to learn new skills and adapt to change.** These qualities are powerful tools in navigating the complex realities of low vision—and in building a life that remains rich, meaningful, and fulfilling despite the challenges.

For many people, adjusting to vision loss involves more than just practical changes—it becomes a journey of inner transformation. Some find strength and comfort in spiritual or religious beliefs, while others draw meaning from personal philosophies, mindfulness practices, or a sense of connection to something greater than themselves. Whether through prayer, meditation, nature, or reflection, these sources of meaning can offer hope, resilience, and perspective during difficult times. Embracing this inner life can be just as important to healing as any medical or practical support.

In the End...

While the experience of vision loss can be emotionally devastating—and daily life may initially feel overwhelming—it's important to recognize that one can still lead a successful, productive, and fulfilling life.

This journey often unfolds through a step-by-step process of acceptance, adjustment, and adaptation. Individuals who thrive with low vision frequently develop compensatory strategies and embrace assistive technologies that allow them to stay engaged, independent, and capable.

The support of family, friends, professionals, and community resources can make a significant difference in rebuilding confidence and self-esteem. Equally important is learning to advocate for your own needs—whether in healthcare, education, work, or social settings. Speaking up and asking for what you need is not just a right; it's an act of strength.

With time, patience, and the right support system, it is entirely possible to navigate the challenges of low vision—and to live a rich, rewarding life filled with purpose and possibility.

References

1. Parent Center Hub .org. FIND YOUR PARENT CENTER

2. U.S. Equal Employment Opportunity Commission, Fact Sheet: Disability Discrimination. Citation: ADA, Rehabilitation Act, 29 CFR Part 1630

Understanding the Link to Depression and Anxiety

Studies have revealed a significant correlation between disabilities, such as vision loss, and the experience of depression and anxiety. Among the various disabilities, vision loss stands out as one of the most daunting, profoundly affecting daily life and playing a pivotal role in the onset of depression and anxiety. The fear accompanying the onset of vision loss often leads to negative attitudes and challenges in adjusting to a life with disability. Understanding this connection is important for developing effective coping strategies.

The Impact of Vision Loss on Mental Health: How vision loss can affect your life.

When considering the effects of vision loss, it's important to look beyond the physical limitations and recognize the significant toll it can take on mental health. Depression and anxiety are common, yet often overlooked, emotional responses to losing one's sight. These struggles affect people of all ages, from children to older adults, and can remain unacknowledged and untreated.

Depression is more than just sadness. It can range from mild and occasional to severe and persistent. For individuals with vision loss, depressive symptoms are often linked to the emotional weight of losing autonomy, the frustration of adapting to daily challenges, and the isolation that can result from diminished social engagement. While the physical act of losing sight is distressing, it's often the accompanying changes in lifestyle and independence that deepen psychological suffering.

The American Psychiatric Association (1) identifies major depression as having *five* of the following **nine** criteria:

1. Depressed mood such as feeling sad, empty, tearful, or irritable most of the day, nearly every day;

2. Decreased interest or pleasure in most activities, most of each day;

3. Significant weight change (5%) or change in appetite;

4. Change in sleep: Insomnia or increased interest in sleep;

5. Change in activity: restless or lethargic;

6. Fatigue or loss of energy;

7. Feelings of worthlessness or excessive or inappropriate guilt;

8. Find it difficult to think or concentrate or an inability to make decisions; and

9. Thoughts of death or suicide.

I would like to add:

10. Outbursts of anger, irritability, seemingly inappropriate for the situation.

In older adults, vision loss is closely tied to a decline in quality of life. Feelings of diminished self-worth, helplessness, and a perceived loss of control can easily lead to depression and anxiety. This emotional toll doesn't just coexist with vision loss—it can compound its effects, further limiting one's ability to function and engage with the world.

Left unaddressed, this cycle can create a downward spiral in mental and physical health. That's why recognizing and treating depression and anxiety in people with visual impairments is essential. By understanding these emotional challenges, healthcare providers, family members, and caregivers can offer more holistic and compassionate care—supporting not just the eyes, but the whole person. 'It takes a village.'

Prevalence of Depression Among the Visually Impaired

As populations in developed countries grow older, the number of adults experiencing vision impairment is steadily increasing. With this rise comes a concerning trend in mental health: studies show that nearly one-third of adults who have recently lost their vision develop clinical depression. This rate is more than double that of their peers without visual impairments. (2)

The risk is especially high in the early stages of vision loss, when individuals are grappling with sudden changes in independence, identity, and daily functioning. These statistics underscore the urgent need for mental health interventions tailored to the unique emotional challenges faced by the visually impaired.

Risk Factors for Depression:

Several factors increase the likelihood of depression among people experiencing vision loss. Understanding these risks can help guide early intervention and support.

Social Isolation and Living Circumstances
Living alone can significantly increase the risk of depression, particularly when vision loss makes individuals feel like prisoners in their own homes. Fear or insecurity about navigating unfamiliar environments often leads to withdrawal from once-enjoyed activities and relationships. Over time, this isolation can deepen emotional distress and create a sense of disconnection from the outside world.

Financial Strain and Shifting Family Roles
The financial consequences of vision loss can be overwhelming. Some individuals may be forced to leave their jobs, while others face mounting medical expenses or the cost of assistive technologies. These economic pressures often shift financial responsibility to other family members, which can strain relationships and add emotional stress on both sides.

Younger Age at Onset
When vision loss occurs during midlife (ages 40–59), it can be particularly devastating. At this stage, most people are actively involved in careers, raising families, and planning for the future. The sudden onset of vision impairment interrupts these plans and may feel like a premature end to goals and independence, making emotional adjustment more difficult than for those who experience vision loss later in life.

Functional Vision and Perception of Ability
How a person perceives their remaining vision and their ability to function day-to-day plays a significant role in mental well-being. Poor functional vision—not just in a clinical sense, but in how it's experienced—can contribute to frustration, helplessness, and a greater risk of depression. In fact, this

emotional toll can further impair one's ability to use their remaining vision effectively.

Difficulty Accepting Vision Loss
Emotional denial can also become a barrier to psychological adjustment. Some individuals hold onto hope that their vision will return or that a cure is imminent. While hope can be a positive force, persistent denial of one's condition may delay acceptance and the adoption of coping strategies, leaving individuals vulnerable to chronic depression.

Age-Related Macular Degeneration (AMD)
AMD is the most common cause of vision loss among adults over 60 in developed countries. Its gradual but progressive nature can be emotionally taxing, especially when individuals struggle to adjust to diminishing central vision over time. The prevalence of depression in those with AMD underscores the importance of regular mental health screening in this population.

Coexisting Health Conditions
Other physical health problems also increase the risk of depression, particularly when combined with visual impairment. Chronic illnesses, mobility limitations, or pain can compound the emotional burden, further restrict activities and diminishing quality of life. (3)

Anxiety and Vision Loss

Anxiety often walks hand in hand with depression, bringing its own unique set of challenges. Like depression, anxiety can persist over time and take many forms, from constant low-level worry to intense fear and avoidance. It often interferes with behavior, decision-making, and the ability to adapt to new routines.

Even minor anxieties can have a profound impact. Fear of making mistakes—such as pressing the wrong button on a stove or misusing a smartphone—can undermine confidence and discourage independence. This fear of error often leads individuals to avoid learning or using new tools, even when those tools could increase their autonomy.

On a broader level, anxiety can lead to isolation. Apprehension about social situations—fear of being judged, pitied, or misunderstood—often drives people to withdraw. Traveling alone may feel daunting. Embarrassment over missing visual cues, like facial expressions or body language, can contribute to a sense of being "alone in a crowd." When others share visual jokes or gestures that go unnoticed, individuals may feel excluded or uncertain about how they're being perceived. These seemingly small moments can feed a cycle of self-consciousness and withdrawal.

One of the most profound sources of anxiety is the fear of **total blindness**. For many individuals, this fear extends far beyond the loss of visual input—it represents a perceived loss of independence, identity, and control over one's future. Questions arise about personal safety, employment, relationships, and the ability to navigate the world without constant assistance. Even when total blindness is medically unlikely, the uncertainty of disease progression can keep the mind anchored in worst-case scenarios, fueling chronic anxiety.

This fear is often compounded by others' lack of understanding. Because many people with visual impairments still function capably in familiar environments, outsiders may underestimate the difficulty of adapting. This can create pressure to **"pass"** as fully sighted—a concept explored in more detail in another chapter. Failing to meet these perceived expectations, even if only self-imposed, can erode self-esteem and intensify anxiety.

Acknowledging and addressing these anxieties is essential to holistic well-being. Understanding the emotional landscape of vision loss allows for more compassionate care, better coping strategies, and deeper personal resilience.

Depression and Anxiety in Visually Impaired Children

Children with visual impairments often face emotional challenges that are difficult to articulate, especially in the early stages of their development. Their understanding of how they differ from peers may be vague or incomplete, which adds to their confusion and emotional vulnerability.

The early years are foundational for self-perception and identity. How children are treated by the adults around them—especially teachers, caregivers, and family members—can deeply influence their self-image. When adults are overly helpful or unintentionally condescending, the child may begin to see themselves as "slow" or incapable. This can sow seeds of self-doubt and low confidence.

Peer relationships also play a major role. Sighted children may not understand the use of assistive tools such as magnifiers, screen readers, or thick eyeglasses. As a result, teasing or exclusion can occur, leading the visually impaired child to feel isolated or ashamed. Being left out of activities that others take for granted—like sports or visual games—can further erode self-esteem.

Additionally, children are highly attuned to their parents' emotions. While it's natural for parents to worry and seek answers, they may unknowingly project anxiety and fear onto their child. This emotional mirroring can heighten the child's own sense of insecurity or apprehension, making emotional regulation more difficult.

Like adults, children with vision loss may experience persistent sadness, fear, or worry. However, because younger children often lack the vocabulary to describe these emotions, their struggles may appear through behavior or physical symptoms rather than words. It's important for caregivers and professionals to recognize the signs of anxiety and depression early.

Common signs of anxiety in children include: (4)

- Irritability
- Avoidance of school or social activities
- Difficulty sleeping
- Fatigue
- Stomachaches or nausea

Signs of depression may mirror those seen in adults and can include:

- Persistent sadness or low mood
- Reluctance to participate in activities they once enjoyed
- Changes in eating patterns (either increased or decreased appetite)
- Sleep disturbances (sleeping more or less than usual)
- Low energy or restlessness
- Difficulty concentrating
- Low self-esteem or confidence

Recognizing these emotional red flags is a critical step in supporting the mental health of visually impaired children. Early identification and intervention can help foster resilience, emotional strength, and a more positive self-image as they grow.

Supporting Your Visually Impaired Child Through Depression and Anxiety

Life with a visual impairment is not the end of the road. Many blind and visually impaired individuals lead rich, successful lives—pursuing college degrees, building meaningful careers, developing strong relationships, and even competing in the Olympics. These examples serve as powerful reminders of what is possible with encouragement, opportunity, and determination.

As a parent or caregiver, one of the most important things you can do is **empower your child to face challenges with confidence**. Encourage problem-solving and resilience. While it's natural to want to protect and assist, avoid doing everything for them. Excessive help can unintentionally send the message that they are incapable. Instead, offer love, affection, and moral support while promoting independence.

Support your child's social and emotional growth by encouraging friendships and connection. Participation in peer groups, support networks, or recreational activities tailored for visually impaired youth can help build essential social skills and reduce feelings of isolation. These interactions are valuable for developing confidence and coping strategies.

If your child is showing signs of depression or anxiety, don't hesitate to seek professional help. Therapists who specialize in working with children with disabilities—including vision impairment—can provide tools to help your child understand and manage their emotions. Counseling may also help you as a parent gain insight into your child's experience and discover new ways to support their mental health.

By fostering independence, offering emotional support, and building a network of care, you are giving your child the foundation to thrive. With your guidance, they can learn to navigate their world with confidence and embrace a life full of possibility.

Addressing Depression in the Visually Disabled: The Treatment Pathway

Treating depression in the visually disabled community can be challenging as it often goes undetected and untreated. There is a reluctance to acknowledge

73

depression, perhaps due to the stigma surrounding mental health issues, or the misconception that it's an inevitable part of aging with no definitive cure. Some individuals may find it difficult to seek help if they deny their feelings, dismissing them as just temporary sadness. Some individuals may feel that seeking help is a sign of weakness, leading to prolonged suffering.

Successful treatment typically involves a comprehensive approach, starting with a low vision evaluation conducted by a specialized professional such as a low vision specialist, often an optometrist. Additionally, a rehabilitation therapist—usually an occupational therapist trained in low vision rehabilitation—can provide valuable assistance. In some cases, a psychiatrist trained in counseling individuals with disabilities may also play an important role in developing a holistic treatment plan. This multidisciplinary approach ensures that the individual receives the tailored support needed to address their depression effectively.

Psychotherapy and Family Counseling

Individual psychotherapy provides a safe space to explore feelings of grief, frustration, and isolation. A trained therapist can help the person adjust to life with a disability, manage social interactions, and cope with the emotional weight of others' perceptions.

Equally important is the role of family counseling. The dynamics within a household often shift when a member becomes visually impaired. Tensions may arise, whether from caregiving burdens, unspoken fears, or changes in roles. Joint counseling sessions can help families navigate these transitions together, promoting better communication, shared understanding, and emotional healing for everyone involved.

In the End;

Depression and anxiety are all too common among individuals with visual impairments, yet they often go undetected and untreated. In the process of adjusting to vision loss, mental health concerns can take a backseat—overlooked under the assumption that treating the physical impairment alone will be enough. This oversight can leave people feeling unheard, isolated, and emotionally overwhelmed.

It's important to **advocate for your mental health needs**. If counseling or support services are not offered, seek them out. There is no shame in asking for help. Depression is a well-recognized consequence of both acquired disability and aging—and addressing it is an important step toward reclaiming emotional balance and a fulfilling quality of life.

Your mental health matters just as much as your physical health. Seeking support is not a sign of weakness—it's an act of strength. You deserve compassionate care, both for your vision and your emotional well-being. Reaching out is a courageous step toward a brighter, more hopeful tomorrow.

He is a wise man who does not grieve for the things which he has not, but rejoices for those which he has.

Epictetus (Greek Stoic philosopher)

References

1. **American Psychiatric Association,** Psychiatry.org - What Is Depression? Depression > What si Depression?

2. Zhang X, Bullard KM, Cotch MF, Wilson MR, Rovner BW, McGwin G Jr, Owsley C, Barker L, Crews JE, Saaddine JB. Association between depression and functional vision loss in persons 20 years of age or older in the United States, NHANES 2005-2008. JAMA Ophthalmol. 2013 May;131(5):573-81. doi: 10.1001/jamaophthalmol.2013.2597. PMID: 23471505; PMCID: PMC3772677.

3. Nollett C, Ryan B, Bray N, Bunce C, Casten R, Edwards RT, Gillespie D, Smith DJ, Stanford M, Margrain TH. Depressive symptoms in people with vision impairment: a cross-sectional study to identify who is most at risk. BMJ Open. 2019 Jan 17;9(1):e026163. doi: 10.1136/bmjopen-2018-026163. PMID: 30782756; PMCID: PMC6340416.

4. Anxiety and Depression in Children, Centers for Disease Control, Children's Mental Health, www.cdc.gov.

Why the Visually Impaired Refuse Low Vision Aids

Refusing low vision aids most commonly involves the psycho-social hurdles of denial, depression, resistance to change, self-image, failure of previous experiences, and cost. To truly empower ourselves, we must confront the psychological and social barriers that hinder us.

Accepting our disabilities, **adjusting** our lifestyles, and utilizing tools are important steps towards **adaptation**. The quality of life is dependent on your capability to adapt.

Do you see yourself or someone you know with any of the following limitations?

1. Denial

Some individuals genuinely believe they do not need visual aids. If they struggle to see something, they blame the size of the print or the design of the object rather than acknowledge any personal vision loss. Others blame the doctor, convinced their prescription is incorrect or that something is wrong with their glasses.

For many, using a low vision aid feels like admitting to having a disability—something they are not ready to accept. This denial runs deep. No amount of persuasion may change their mind, and they may even give up once-enjoyed activities, like reading, rather than acknowledge the need for help.

2. Depression

Some individuals experiencing vision loss become overwhelmed by grief and hopelessness. They have given up—not just on visual aids, but on the idea that things could improve. Motivation is low, and they are not yet ready to adjust their thinking or embrace change.

For them, using a low vision aid may feel like further surrender to their disability, reinforcing a sense of loss rather than offering hope. In these cases, psychosocial counseling can be an essential step toward helping them process their emotions, regain motivation, and begin moving forward.

3. Resistance to New Things

For some, resistance to low vision aids stems from a personality trait—a general reluctance to try anything unfamiliar. They may assume the devices will be too complicated to use or believe they lack the energy or mental bandwidth to learn something new.

Fortunately, with the right encouragement and support, many discover that low vision aids are not as difficult to master as they feared—and that the benefits are well worth the effort.

4. Self-Image

For some individuals, avoiding low vision aids is closely tied to a desire to appear "normal." They may fear that using a device will draw unwanted attention or prompt uncomfortable questions from others.

There is often a deep concern that using visual aids will cause others to label them as blind—an identity they may not relate to and one that can feel threatening to their self-esteem. The stigma, whether real or perceived, can be a powerful barrier to acceptance.

5. Previous Experience

Many people reject low vision aids because of a disappointing past experience. Perhaps they tried a magnifier from a department store, or one given to them by a well-meaning family member. They used it briefly, found it ineffective, and concluded that these devices simply "don't work."

But that quick trial—under harsh store lighting, using a low-power, general-purpose magnifier—was never a fair test. Most store-bought aids are not tailored for long-term use or specific visual tasks, and they often lack the optical quality or strength needed for meaningful assistance. Without proper assessment and guidance, it's easy to dismiss the very tools that could help.

6.. Cost

Cost is often a major reason people refuse low vision aids. Throughout my career as an optometrist, I was frequently surprised by the choices people made—someone might spend hundreds on a designer handbag but hesitate to invest in the glasses they wear every day. I also saw parents take their child to Disney World, yet balk at spending a reasonable amount on high-quality eyewear for that same child.

There's no denying that specialized visual aids can be expensive. But like any tool, their value must be weighed against their potential to improve daily functioning and independence. This is why a low vision evaluation is so important. It allows you to receive expert guidance, try out various devices in a controlled setting, and make informed choices—possibly saving you from making a costly mistake down the line.

Those That Have Devices and Just Don't Use Them

In my experience with low vision patients, I've often presented them with a range of low vision devices and technologies that have the potential to transform their lives, reigniting their interests in activities they once loved. However, despite initial interest, many of these patients find themselves lacking the motivation to fully embrace these aids. They've settled into a life adjusted to their disability, putting their hobbies and interests on the back burner due to the perceived difficulty of adopting new compensatory techniques.

Take quilting, for example. A quilter may need to use a magnifier between their glasses and their needlework, adjust their posture, upgrade lighting at both their sewing station and machine, and learn new ways to cut fabric. The process involves acquiring new tools and, more importantly, the patience to master them. (FYI, here is a good article on 'Quilting Techniques' follow Vision,Career Connect. (1)

So, what sets apart those who persevere and those who give up? **Motivation** plays a significant role. *Are individuals willing to invest the time and effort required to learn new methods?* Generally, younger low vision patients are more open to learning and adapting, while seniors may struggle more with the idea of making significant adjustments.

In some cases, a concept known as **secondary gain** may influence a person's willingness to adapt. Secondary gain refers to the indirect benefits a person may receive as a result of their condition. These can include financial compensation, disability benefits, accommodations at work or school, or even increased attention and support from others. While not necessarily conscious or deliberate, these gains can reduce motivation to pursue greater independence, including the use of low vision aids.

(Secondary gain is discussed in more depth in the chapter: **Why the Visually Impaired Resist Therapy**.)

Another common barrier is lack of **adequate training and reinforcement.** Simply handing someone a device is rarely enough. Without hands-on instruction and follow-up support, many patients forget how to use their devices effectively— or never reach the point of using them to their full potential. In my own practice, I've seen patients benefit tremendously from a brief **refresher course**, which often restores confidence and improves outcomes.

Finally, the perceived usefulness of a device plays a critical role. For example, video magnifiers have revolutionized magnification options for the visually impaired. But if a device is too cumbersome, has a limited visual field, or doesn't align with the user's specific needs—such as reading a newspaper—it may end up collecting dust. That's why device selection must always be tailored to the individual, with careful consideration of their daily tasks and functional goals.

Understanding Those Who Refuse to Use Low Vision Devices

The type and extent of vision loss can greatly influence an individual's openness to using low vision aids. Those with central vision loss—such as from macular degeneration or Stargardt's disease—often respond well to magnification and other adaptive tools. In contrast, individuals with peripheral vision loss, as seen in conditions like glaucoma or retinitis pigmentosa, may find traditional magnifiers less helpful and face greater difficulty with adaptation. (2)

This variability underscores the importance of personalized guidance from low vision specialists and therapists. Trial-and-error methods or well-meaning gifts from loved ones rarely lead to success. In fact, trying devices that don't work can be frustrating and discouraging, reinforcing a sense of helplessness.

Understanding the emotional landscape of vision loss is essential. While cost is a tangible factor, most resistance to low vision aids is psychological—rooted in grief, fear, frustration, or self-image. Often, a lack of knowledge and experience adds to the hesitation.

That's why it's so important to approach these situations with empathy, patience, and a commitment to education. By addressing both the emotional and practical barriers, we can support individuals in overcoming resistance and embracing tools that can significantly enhance their independence and quality of life.

In the End...

The challenge of unused low vision devices is rarely due to a single issue. It often arises from a combination of factors: lack of motivation, inadequate training, and poor device fit. Overcoming these barriers requires more than just access to tools—it takes a willingness to learn, professional support, and thoughtful, individualized device selection.

When these needs are met with empathy and expertise, individuals with low vision are far more likely to embrace these aids and rediscover activities they once enjoyed. In doing so, they can improve their independence, confidence, and overall quality of life.

> *It is hard to fail, but it is worse never*
>
> *to have tried to succeed.*
>
> **Theodore Roosevelt**

References

1. Quilting, American Printing House for the Blind, Career Connect

2. Dougherty BE, Kehler KB, Jamara R, Patterson N, Valenti D, Vera-Diaz FA. Abandonment of low-vision devices in an outpatient population. Optom Vis Sci. 2011 Nov;88(11):1283-7. doi: 10.1097/OPX.0b013e31822a61e7. PMID: 21822160; PMCID: PMC3204005.

Why the Visually Impaired Resist Therapy

Resistance to therapy among individuals with visual impairments often stems from emotional and psychological challenges, including fear, anxiety, depression, and, at times, the unconscious benefits of remaining dependent—a concept known as **secondary gain**.

Rehabilitation therapy offers individuals the opportunity to make the most of their remaining vision. It combines the use of optical aids, non-optical devices, and assistive technologies with training in compensatory strategies. The goal is to help people with low vision achieve greater independence in education, employment, and daily life.

Successful rehabilitation is a collaborative process involving eye care professionals, therapists, and the individual with vision loss. Yet, its success ultimately depends on the individual's readiness to participate—something often complicated by psychological and social barriers.

How *Depression* Affects the Rehabilitation Process

Among the many challenges in adapting to visual impairment, depression often stands as the primary obstacle. Numerous studies have shown a strong association between vision loss and depression, especially in older adults. As noted in *JAMA Ophthalmology*, "vision loss is among the most common chronic conditions associated with depression in old age." (1)

The emotional toll of losing vision frequently triggers a cascade of frustration, fear, and anxiety, leaving individuals feeling helpless and diminished in self-worth. As the outlook on life darkens, the burden of living with visual impairment can lead to deep despair and clinical depression.

Recovery from this emotional state is not always straightforward. For some, the path out of depression is long and uncertain. Depression often exists within a complex web of factors—age, coexisting medical conditions, social support, living circumstances, financial stress, and even substance abuse.

Recognizing depression is the essential first step toward adaptation and rehabilitation. Effective vision rehabilitation must address these psychosocial needs alongside functional training. Referrals for counseling and emotional support should be an integral part of the rehabilitation process, not an afterthought.

Without such support, feelings of helplessness, reduced independence, and poor self-image can become major barriers to progress, hindering the development of adaptive skills and limiting overall success in therapy.

How *Fear* can Make the Visually Impaired Resistant to Therapy

Fear—both large and small—can create powerful barriers to therapy for individuals with visual impairments. Major fears often involve concerns about safety and independence: navigating busy streets, maneuvering through unfamiliar office buildings or airports, or functioning without being able to see important details. There's also the persistent worry: *"Am I going to make a mistake?"*

Smaller, yet deeply felt fears often center around the possibility of making mistakes that appear careless or unintelligent to others. Individuals with low vision may fear being perceived as incompetent if they misread a label, fumble with unfamiliar devices, or ask for clarification. The dread of seeming "dim-witted" or incapable—not because of a lack of ability, but because of how their vision loss affects their actions—can be humiliating. This fear can quietly undermine confidence, making people reluctant to try new tools, attempt daily tasks, or participate in therapy where mistakes are part of the learning process.

Technology can also be intimidating. Low vision aids often come with unfamiliar buttons, confusing features, and unclear instructions. When devices feel unintuitive, the **fear of failure** or embarrassment increases. Similarly, adapting tasks at home or at work—especially in the kitchen or a professional setting—can feel overwhelming. People may fear making mistakes, appearing incompetent, or being unable to keep up.

These fears, whether related to judgment, technology, or daily functioning, can discourage participation in rehabilitation. Addressing them with patience, reassurance, and practical instruction is vital to helping individuals move forward.

While fear often stems from unfamiliar tasks or tools, anxiety is more closely tied to how others might respond. These emotional hurdles often go hand-in-hand, making it difficult for individuals with low vision to step outside their comfort zones and fully engage in rehabilitation.

Why *Anxiety* Causes Avoidance

Anxiety tends to thrive in social situations, especially those involving acquaintances or strangers. While interactions with close friends or family may feel safe, stepping into unfamiliar environments often triggers deep worry about how one will be perceived.

While fear often arises in **response to specific, external challenges**—like using unfamiliar tools or navigating public spaces—anxiety tends to be more internal. It's rooted in **social perceptions, self-consciousness, and emotional vulnerability**.

For individuals with low vision, anxious thoughts may include: *Do they understand what low vision really means? Will I have to explain my condition again? Will they see me as the person I was before—or pity me, treat me differently, or assume I'm less capable?* This ongoing pressure to clarify a hidden disability can be emotionally draining.

One particularly distressing aspect of vision loss is the ambiguity it presents to others. Someone may be 'legally blind' yet still have functional vision, leading to repeated misunderstandings. The anxiety of being misjudged—or misunderstood—can make social participation feel risky.

As a result, avoidance often becomes a coping mechanism. The internal dialogue shifts to: *"If I avoid this situation, I won't have to explain myself. I won't risk embarrassment. Since I can't see well, maybe it's safer not to participate at all."* Over time, this mindset can lead to increasing isolation and disengagement from rehabilitation.

When Lack of Goals Leads to Resistance

One often-overlooked reason individuals resist therapy is the absence of clear, meaningful goals. Without a vision for what rehabilitation can help them achieve, it's easy to feel directionless—or even question the point of therapy at all.

When therapy is presented in vague or overwhelming terms, anxiety tends to increase. People may think, *"What am I really working toward?"*, or *"Will this even help me function better?"* This lack of clarity can result in avoidance, missed appointments, or half-hearted engagement.

Without defined objectives—like learning to use a magnifier for reading books, mastering a screen reader for employment, or safely navigating public transportation—the process can seem abstract and unmotivating. Therapy may feel like a reminder of limitations rather than a pathway to progress.

Helping individuals identify concrete, achievable goals transforms therapy from a source of stress into a tool for reclaiming independence. But when those goals are absent or unclear, resistance is a natural response.

The Phenomenon of Secondary Gain

Secondary gain is a psychological concept that refers to the subtle benefits a person may experience as a result of their disability. While vision loss brings undeniable challenges, it can also lead to unintended advantages—social, emotional, or practical—that influence how someone engages with rehabilitation.

These benefits can range from small conveniences, like having others take over daily tasks, to more significant outcomes such as reduced responsibilities or access to financial compensation. Over time, these advantages can create unconscious incentives to remain dependent, even when greater independence is possible.

Consider an example: An individual with central vision loss struggles with tasks like reading mail, paying bills, or using kitchen appliances. They share these difficulties with family and friends, who respond with kindness and eagerness to help. While their vision is still partially functional, the individual begins to appreciate the extra support and attention. Gradually, they may find themselves relying more on others—not necessarily out of need, but because of the comfort and care it brings.

This is not a matter of deliberate deception. Rather, it's a subtle psychological trap: the more support they receive, the less motivated they may feel to pursue tools or training that could restore independence.

Intervention can shift this dynamic. With the help of an optometrist or occupational therapist trained in adaptive strategies, the individual discovers new ways to manage daily tasks—restoring a sense of control. Yet this shift may feel threatening to established roles. Family and friends, having stepped in as caregivers, may begin to pull back support once the individual starts regaining self-sufficiency. The result can be emotionally complex for everyone involved.

Understanding secondary gain is key to overcoming this barrier. Recognizing the unconscious motivations at play—both for the individual and their support network—can open the door to more balanced, empowering rehabilitation.

Secondary gain can take many forms:

Secondary gain can manifest in a variety of ways—often subtly, and frequently without the person even realizing it. Some examples include:

- Using the disability to reduce or avoid work responsibilities.
- Receiving increased sympathy or attention from others.
- Opting out of tasks they find unpleasant, such as cooking, household chores, or childcare.
- Avoiding social engagements or obligations, leading to a pattern of self-isolation.
- Transferring responsibilities to others, fostering a deeper sense of dependency.
- Strengthening emotional bonds through increased care-taking from family and friends.
- In some cases, using the disability to assert control in relationships or influence outcomes.

It's important to note that *not all* individuals with vision loss experience or act on secondary gains—and when they do, it's rarely intentional. In many cases, the person is unaware that these patterns have developed. A perceptive family member, counselor, or vision rehabilitation specialist may be the first to recognize how these dynamics are affecting the rehabilitation process.

Acknowledging secondary gain is not about blame. It's about understanding the hidden psychological roadblocks that may slow progress or lead to stalled motivation. At the same time, it's essential to consider other possible contributing factors—such as underlying medical conditions or mental health concerns—that may mimic or amplify the effects of secondary gain.

By recognizing these complex emotional layers, therapists and support teams can offer more compassionate, effective guidance—encouraging individuals to pursue greater independence without fear of losing support or connection.

Understanding the subtle ways secondary gain manifests is only part of the picture. What's equally important is recognizing how these unconscious rewards can directly interfere with progress. When the benefits of dependency feel more emotionally rewarding—or safer—than the uncertain path toward independence, the motivation to adapt can quietly erode.

Secondary Gain Can Reduce Motivation to Adapt

Adapting to a disability often requires significant effort. It means learning new techniques, navigating unfamiliar tools, and accepting uncomfortable change. Yet for some individuals, the perceived benefits of vision loss—such as attention, concern, or exemption from certain responsibilities—can make the status quo feel preferable.

In these cases, even the most well-designed rehabilitation programs may be met with quiet resistance. While doctors and specialists promote tools that increase independence, the person receiving care may feel conflicted. Using a magnifier or assistive device might not just represent progress—it could threaten a valued source of connection or care.

When these unconscious dynamics are at play, motivation to engage with therapy may wane. Progress stalls—not because the person doesn't want to improve, but because improvement comes with emotional trade-offs that must be acknowledged and addressed with sensitivity.

In the End... Getting Help

Resistance to therapy among individuals with visual impairments is often rooted in complex emotional and psychological factors, including fear, anxiety, depression, and the influence of secondary gain. These barriers can make adaptation feel daunting—but they are not insurmountable.

Mental health professionals play a vital role in helping individuals recognize and work through these challenges. With the right support, those experiencing vision loss can better manage the emotional toll, improve interpersonal relationships, and begin to embrace strategies that foster independence.

Overcoming resistance to therapy is not only about learning to live with vision loss—it's about reclaiming confidence, rediscovering purpose, and building a fulfilling life.

Your life does not get better by chance, it gets better by change.

Jim Rohn

Reference

1. Zhang X, Bullard KM, Cotch MF, Wilson MR, Rovner BW, McGwin G Jr, Owsley C, Barker L, Crews JE, Saaddine JB. Association between depression and functional vision loss in persons 20 years of age or older in the United States, NHANES 2005-2008. JAMA Ophthalmol. 2013 May;131(5):573-81. doi: 10.1001/jamaophthalmol.2013.2597. PMID: 23471505; PMCID: PMC3772677.

Pretending Not to be Visually Impaired: Passing with a Disability

Individuals with vision impairment often adopt behaviors and tactics to hide their disability, striving to blend in and appear "normal." This is facilitated by the fact that vision impairment is often categorized as an "invisible" condition.

What is Passing?

"Passing" in the context of disability refers to the intentional act of concealing one's disability. It involves individuals with disabilities attempting to appear as if they do not have a disability, especially in social situations. This can involve hiding behaviors or characteristics associated with their disability to blend in with able-bodied individuals.

Vision impairment is often considered "invisible" because it may not be immediately apparent to others when interacting with someone with this disability. There are typically no outward signs of vision loss unless a person exhibits specific low vision behaviors, such as holding objects very close, tilting their head, excessive blinking, or eye movements that appear unfocused or exaggerated.

Passing may seem deceptive or dishonest to some, as individuals are essentially pretending to be able-bodied when they are not. However, for many with vision impairment, the decision to pass as fully sighted is deeply personal and often driven by emotional reasons.

Living in a world between the blind and the sighted, those with visual impairment often use passing as a form of self-defense. It allows them to create a façade of normalcy, helping to protect their social acceptance and preserve their psychological well-being.

Why the Visually Impaired Conceal Their Disability

Social Pressure: The social stigma attached to the term "disability" can subconsciously compel those with invisible disabilities to conceal their condition, aiming to sidestep the negative social implications of deviating from what is considered "normal."

Lack of Understanding: Many individuals without visual impairments may not fully comprehend what "low vision" entails. Social norms often equate disability with a perceived lack of capability, extending beyond just the ability to see. Vision impairment is sometimes mistakenly equated with blindness or even intellectual disability.

They may find it is just easier to pretend. Openly identifying themselves as disabled, means opening up the "I can't see, but I'm not blind" litany.

Ease of Passing: At times, "passing" as sighted is simply easier than delving into detailed explanations of personal limitations. This approach helps avoid the use of terms like "disabled" or "impaired," which can steer conversations into uncomfortable or negative territory. Responding to such terms, listeners may exhibit patronizing attitudes or expressions of pity. To sidestep these reactions, visually impaired individuals may choose to pass as sighted for their own comfort and that of those around them.

Persistent Biases: Despite advancements in legislation and changing social attitudes toward disabilities, personal biases still linger, affecting how individuals perceive and react to disability. These lingering biases contribute to the inclination to conceal one's visual impairment in social settings.

Self-Image: For those newly experiencing visual loss, acceptance of their low vision may still be an ongoing journey. Choosing to remain silent about their disability can be a defense mechanism to uphold feelings of self-worth and a sense of normalcy.

Social Stigma and Self-Esteem: The societal stigma surrounding disabilities can lead to negative self-perceptions among the visually impaired. They may struggle with feelings of low self-esteem, perceiving themselves as "less-than" others.

Our self-perception is often influenced by how others perceive us. By not openly declaring "I am visually impaired," individuals with disabilities aim to maintain equal standing with their peers. This is an attempt to resist being solely defined by their disability.

Privacy Concerns: Disclosing one's disability and sharing personal details can feel invasive. Many visually impaired individuals view their visual status as private information, to be disclosed on a need-to-know basis.

Shame and Embarrassment: Past experiences with impaired vision that led to embarrassment or feelings of inferiority can result in a deep sense of shame. Others seem superior because they can see more quickly, react appropriately, and are queued into nuances of social interaction.

All of these seemingly small details of social interaction work due to better visual acuity. Facial recognition, facial expression, and visual jokes are missed by those with low vision leaving them to feel left out and embarrassed. Passing as sighted becomes a method of hiding what they perceive as a weakness or inadequacy.

Social Exclusion and Fear: Fear plays a significant role in this dynamic:

- **Fear of loss of social acceptance.**
- **Fear of being marginalized or excluded and loss of social status**.
- **Fear of losing a job** because of assumptions made by others who do not understand.
- **Fear of Self-Realization:** Admitting to oneself that they are not "normal" can be a daunting and fearful prospect.
- **Fear of Social Judgment:** The anxiety of having to explain their visual impairment in detail, knowing others will pass judgment.
- **Fear of being singled out or treated differently** due to their disability.

In navigating these complex emotions and societal pressures, visually impaired individuals often find themselves balancing between maintaining their privacy, preserving their self-image, and navigating a world that often fails to fully understand their experiences.

How Children Learn to Pass

Pretending to See: Children often adjust their behavior to match what they believe others expect of them, sometimes pretending to see more or less than they actually can.

Parental Influence: Children are keen observers of their parents' attitudes and fears. They quickly pick up on the concern surrounding their visual impairment, learning that not seeing what others see is viewed as a problem. To gain approval and avoid worry, children may give false responses, pretending to see things they actually can't. The parent's relief and positive reinforcement become a reward for their pretense.

Avoidance and Ignorance: Parents may sometimes choose to ignore the issue, perhaps due to difficulty in facing the reality of having a visually impaired child. This avoidance communicates to the child that their visual disability is something to be disregarded, contributing to their learning to "pass."

Negative Attention in School: As school-age children, they quickly learn that being different can attract negative attention from peers. Other children may not always be kind or understanding, leading to feelings of exclusion and loneliness.

Treatment and Bullying: Disabled children may be treated as "special," often being segregated from other children and excluded from certain activities due to accessibility challenges. They might also be infantilized, that is, treated more childishly than their sighted peers. This difference in treatment can make them targets for bullying, which can be deeply upsetting and isolating.

Academic Impact: In attempting to pass as normal and avoid negative attention, children may also avoid asking for necessary help. This can result in falling behind academically, as their reluctance to seek assistance hampers their learning progress.

These experiences of social exclusion, bullying, and the pressure to conform to societal norms can have profound effects on a child's development and self-esteem. As they navigate these challenges, children with visual disabilities often learn to hide their disability as a means of coping with the complexities of their social environment.

How Parents Can Help

Parents play an important role in shaping how a child understands and manages their visual impairment. One of the most powerful things a parent can do is to foster open, nonjudgmental communication. Instead of rewarding pretense—whether knowingly or not—parents can gently encourage honesty by creating a safe space for their child to talk about what they truly see and feel. Asking open-ended questions, listening without correction, and validating their experiences helps children feel accepted just as they are.

It's also essential for parents to model healthy attitudes toward disability. When a parent openly acknowledges their child's challenges without fear or shame, the child learns that having a visual impairment is not something to hide or be embarrassed about. Advocating for accommodations in school, encouraging the use of assistive devices, and celebrating the child's efforts and abilities—rather than solely focusing on limitations—helps children build self-confidence. When parents approach vision loss with acceptance, resilience, and hope, children are far less likely to feel the need to pass as sighted.

The Consequences of Pretending to be Normal

Social Awkwardness: When others are unaware of the limitations faced by someone concealing their visual impairment, the visually impaired individual may appear socially awkward. Due to their low vision, they might struggle to recognize faces, interpret facial expressions, and grasp nonverbal cues essential for social interaction. This can lead them to appear distracted or unresponsive in social situations.

Discomfort and Embarrassment: Admitting to not being able to see adequately after concealing it for some time can be uncomfortable and embarrassing. Those who were unaware may feel suspicious upon learning this information, wondering why it was kept hidden.

Difficulty Navigating Social Situations: Navigating social situations with a visual impairment is inherently challenging. This challenge is compounded when others fail to understand the social mistakes that might occur, mistakes not typically made by those with normal vision. Consequently, visually impaired individuals may withdraw from social interactions, leading to feelings of depression and anxiety.

Employment Challenges: Concealing visual impairment from potential employers can pose significant challenges. Passing as sighted may seem like a way to bypass personal biases that some employers have against hiring disabled individuals. Despite legislation aimed at preventing discrimination, it unfortunately still exists.

However, nondisclosure often comes at a cost. When an employee hides their visual impairment, they may forgo **reasonable accommodations** that would allow them to perform their job more effectively and safely. Tasks may take longer, errors may increase, and unnecessary stress can build as the individual expends energy compensating rather than working efficiently. Over time, this constant effort to conceal limitations can lead to fatigue, anxiety, and reduced job satisfaction. (For more information on employment with a disability, see the chapter on The Americans with Disabilities Act and Low Vision.)

Risk of Errors and Job Loss: The fear of being "found out" may discourage asking for help or clarification, increasing the risk of mistakes or misunderstandings. In some cases, performance may be unfairly judged as inadequate, when in reality it reflects a lack of appropriate accommodations rather than a lack of ability.

Opportunity for Education and Awareness: Revealing one's limitations is not just about personal acceptance; it's also an opportunity to educate others. Just as the LGBTQ community has brought awareness and acceptance to their experiences, those with disabilities can also benefit from greater understanding. It's important for others to realize that individuals with impairments are simply a **different form of normal**, deserving of respect, understanding, and the accommodations necessary to thrive.

In the End....

Passing with a visual impairment presents numerous challenges, from social awkwardness to employment uncertainties. The decision to conceal one's disability is often driven by social pressures and fear of stigma. However, there can be consequences leading to discomfort, social difficulties, and missed opportunities for accommodations.

Revealing one's limitations can promote understanding and empathy, fostering a society that values inclusivity. By supporting individuals with visual impairments, we can create a world where everyone can thrive.

Understanding Eye Strain and Headaches in Low Vision: Causes and Solutions

Why Are People with Low Vision Susceptible to Eye Strain and Headaches?

Eye strain and headaches in individuals with low vision often arise from a combination of visual, physical, and mental stressors. These symptoms aren't just due to poor eyesight—they stem from the adaptations required to function with limited vision.

People with low vision frequently:

- Use high levels of magnification,
- Work at closer-than-normal distances,
- Make repeated screen and head movements,
- Use eccentric viewing techniques due to central vision loss

.

It's not merely a matter of declining vision; new obstacles emerge in adapting to the "new normal." Learning to utilize assistive devices and compensatory techniques becomes essential for improved vision. However, it's common for individuals to experience eyestrain and headaches as they adjust. Consequently, these symptoms may lead to reluctance in using adaptive devices and a tendency to avoid tasks like reading, which is particularly problematic for students and professionals.

The widespread accessibility and convenience of computers have rendered them almost indispensable for many visually impaired. However, prolonged periods of screen time can lead to Digital Eye Strain (DES).

Digital Eye Strain and Low Vision

The increasing reliance on digital devices presents additional challenges. Prolonged screen use, particularly with LED backlit displays, can lead to Digital Eye Strain (DES)—also known as Computer Vision Syndrome (CVS). While DES affects many users, it disproportionately impacts those with low vision because of their unique viewing behaviors.

Common DES Symptoms:

- Eye fatigue or heaviness
- Headaches
- Burning, redness, or tearing
- Blurred or double vision
- Neck, shoulder, or back pain
- Increased light sensitivity
- Difficulty concentrating or staying alert

Additional Symptoms Experienced by Those with Low Vision:

- Motion sickness, and
- A sense of muscular strain around the eyes from prolonged effort.

Those with low vision use the technology differently from others because they use magnification, a closer working distance, and more screen movement.

Physical and Mental Contributors to Strain

Eye strain and headaches can stem from various factors, often a combination of visual, physical, and mental stresses.

For individuals grappling with low vision, everyday tasks can become more challenging and time-consuming. While the mental stress of school or work is something many can relate to, it's magnified for those balancing the added complexities of utilizing adaptive techniques and assistive devices to complete tasks. When headaches and eyestrain are added to the equation due to optical and physical adaptations, the mental stress of "seeing" can hinder concentration and comprehension.

Physical stress manifests in how the body adjusts to accommodate digital or assistive technology usage. Some positions required are unnatural:

- Hunching over devices or holding magnifiers at awkward angles
- Leaning forward to see screens or printed text
- Tensing neck and shoulder muscles for prolonged periods

Over time, these unnatural postures and muscular overuse can trigger tension headaches and musculoskeletal discomfort, further compounding the problem.

Strategies to Prevent and Reduce Eyestrain and Headaches

Eye strain and headaches associated with low vision and modern digital technology are multifaceted, with causes varying by individual, assistive technology used, and environmental factors. Here is a step-by-step approach:

1. Consult with an optometrist or low vision specialist to obtain the **optimal eyeglass prescription** (if needed) and select a low vision assistive device tailored to your tasks. The difference between over-the-counter reading glasses and prescription glasses is substantial; improper power selection or mismatched prescriptions for each eye can lead to eyestrain and headaches. You may select a power that is too strong or too-weak. Also, not all eyes are equal. The lenses of common store-bought glasses are both the same power. While the prescription for your eyes may differ from the left eye to right eye. If not properly balanced, this can cause eyestrain and headaches.

2. Determine the **most comfortable magnification level** and the best method to achieve it. Optical devices require a close working distance, but you should avoid hunching forward or squinting while reading. If using low vision digital devices like video magnifiers, seek guidance from your low vision specialist for optimal selection.

3. **Explore options** such as short-wavelength-blocking eyeglass lenses or computer screen filters to alleviate eyestrain associated with digital devices. Blue light-blocking lenses and software applications like Apple's "Night Shift," Android's "Twilight," or Microsoft's "Night light" can reduce blue light exposure.

4. **Address other eye issues** like burning, dry, or watery eyes by consulting an eye doctor for a dry eye evaluation. Simple strategies like remembering to blink regularly or following the 20/20/20 rule (taking a 20-second break every 20 minutes to look 20 feet away) can help alleviate symptoms.

5. **Assess the lighting and glare sources** in your environment. Lighting that is too bright or too dim can exacerbate visual strain, while shiny or glossy surfaces and computer screens can cause reflections that increase eye fatigue and discomfort.

6. Pay attention to the **ergonomics** of your work setup. Workspace ergonomics refers to arranging your work area so your body, head, and eyes are properly aligned, reducing physical strain and visual fatigue while improving comfort and efficiency.

Head, neck, and shoulder pain may signal that your workspace needs adjustment. Your chair, desk height, and the position of reading materials or digital devices should allow you to maintain a relaxed, upright posture with your head and neck in a neutral position. Screens and reading materials should be positioned directly in front of you at a comfortable distance to avoid excessive bending, twisting, or leaning forward. Prolonged hunching over digital or low vision devices can increase muscle tension, contribute to headaches, and worsen eyestrain; small ergonomic adjustments can significantly improve comfort and visual endurance.

Ergonomic Quick-Check Checklist for Reducing Eyestrain and Headaches

- My chair supports my lower back, and my feet rest flat on the floor or a footrest
- My head and neck remain upright and relaxed—not bent forward or tilted down
- My reading material or screen is positioned directly in front of me
- I do not need to hunch, lean, or squint to see my task clearly
- The viewing distance feels comfortable and does not strain my neck or eyes
- Frequently used items are within easy reach
- Lighting is adequate and adjustable without glare or reflections
- I take regular breaks to stretch, change posture, and rest my eyes

Eccentric Viewing: A Helpful but Straining Technique

Eccentric viewing is a technique used by individuals with low vision to utilize their remaining vision for various tasks, such as reading, writing, or viewing distant objects. Those with low vision who have impaired central vision due to conditions such as macular degeneration, Stargardt's disease, or diabetic retinopathy, benefit from this technique.

Instead of relying on central vision, eccentric viewing involves training oneself to use a peripheral area of the retina called the **preferred retinal locus**. This is a specific spot adjacent to the central blind spot where vision may be clearer or less affected by the visual impairment. By shifting their gaze away from the center and using this peripheral area, individuals with low vision can make better use of their remaining functional vision.

However, this requires keeping the eyes in an unnatural position for extended periods. Over time, eccentric viewing can lead to:
- Eye fatigue
- Muscle tension
- Headaches
- Reduced stamina for tasks like reading

Despite the physical toll, eccentric viewing can significantly improve independence. With professional training and pacing, many users find it a worthwhile adaptation that improves quality of life. There is a discussion about eccentric viewing in the chapter on *Low Vision Training: Relearning to See*, pg. 34-35.)

In the End...

Eye strain and headaches are common but manageable concerns for people with low vision. They reflect the physical, visual, and emotional labor required to adapt to a world designed for the fully sighted. Understanding the causes—and implementing supportive strategies—can greatly reduce discomfort, improve performance, and encourage continued use of low vision tools and techniques. Support from vision specialists, appropriate technologies, and thoughtful environmental adjustments can help individuals not only cope but thrive.

Vision Loss and Memory:

Understanding the Connection

Vision plays a vital role in how we take in, process, and remember information. When someone experiences vision loss, their ability to form visual memories—such as recognizing faces, recalling locations, or identifying objects—can be disrupted. This isn't necessarily due to memory loss itself, but rather because the visual information needed to form these memories is either missing or incomplete.

Additionally, people with vision impairment may participate less in visually engaging activities, such as reading, observing their surroundings, or interacting with visual media. This reduction in sensory stimulation may, over time, affect cognitive health. However, it's important to note that vision impairment by itself *does not* directly cause memory loss or dementia. Instead, it may contribute to changes in cognitive function through indirect pathways such as social withdrawal, reduced physical activity, or emotional stress.

Understanding the Brain-Visual Memory Connection

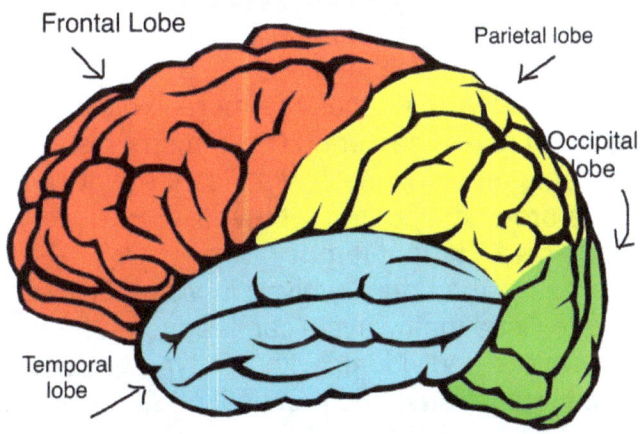

Vision and memory are deeply intertwined, both functionally and neurologically. Much of what we remember is influenced by what we see, and the brain relies on visual input to help form, store, and retrieve memories.

- **Visual Information Processing:**
  The occipital lobe, located at the back of the brain, is responsible for processing visual information. Once visual data is interpreted, it is relayed to other regions—such as the temporal and parietal lobes—where it can be encoded and stored as memory. If visual input is limited or distorted, as in vision impairment, the formation of accurate visual memories can be compromised.
- **Spatial Memory and Navigation:**
  Visual cues—like landmarks, pathways, and environmental details—are important for spatial awareness and navigation. Good vision helps individuals form mental maps of their surroundings, enabling them to remember locations and move through space confidently. When these visual cues are diminished, navigating new or even familiar environments becomes more cognitively demanding. (1)
- **Attention and Focus:**
  Attention plays a vital role in memory formation. Vision guides our focus, allowing us to zero in on relevant stimuli and filter out distractions. People with intact vision typically find it easier to attend to important information, which improves encoding and recall. In contrast, visual impairment can fragment attention, making memory formation more difficult. (3)
- **Perceptual Learning:**
  Perceptual learning refers to the brain's ability to improve the interpretation of sensory input through repetition and experience. For visual information, this involves recognizing patterns, faces, or objects more efficiently over time. This process strengthens visual memory and is closely linked to activity in the brain's visual regions. (2)
- **Emotion and Memory:**
  Emotionally charged experiences are more likely to be remembered, and vision plays a key role in capturing these moments. Seeing a loved one's face or witnessing an emotionally significant event can strongly influence how memories are encoded and retrieved. (3)
- **Brain Damage and Visual Memory:**
  Damage to areas of the brain involved in visual processing—such as the occipital lobe or visual pathways—can lead to both visual impairment and memory deficits. Individuals with this type of damage may struggle to form or recall visual memories, even if other cognitive functions remain intact.

How the Brain Adapts After Vision Loss

The brain is not a passive recipient of sensory loss—it actively reorganizes itself in response. When vision is impaired or lost, the brain compensates by reallocating resources to strengthen other senses, a process known as **neuroplasticity**.

Neuroplasticity refers to the brain's ability to reorganize and form new neural connections in response to sensory changes. This adaptation is especially evident in individuals with vision loss. Rather than processing visual input in the traditional way, the brain increases activity in non-visual regions—particularly the **auditory** and **somatosensory** areas—to help the person gather environmental information through sound and touch. (4)

For example, research shows that individuals who are blind or visually impaired often demonstrate enhanced hearing and tactile abilities. The occipital lobe, which typically processes visual input, can become involved in **non-visual tasks**, such as **Braille reading** or **sound localization**, thereby assisting in navigation and spatial awareness. This phenomenon, known as **cross-modal neuroplasticity**, is a key strategy the brain uses to compensate for sensory loss. (5)

In cases of **partial vision loss**, adaptation may look different. People may still rely on residual vision, but they often need to exert greater mental effort to interpret limited or distorted visual information. This extra effort can reduce cognitive efficiency, affecting **attention**, **concentration**, and **task performance**. Difficulties recognizing faces, reading, or orienting in space may stem from both the sensory limitations and the added mental effort involved in processing unclear input.

It's also important to understand that the extent and nature of brain adaptation can vary depending on the individual, the underlying cause of vision loss, the age at which it occurs, and whether it is **or acquired sudden or gradual**, **congenital**. However, across these variables, the brain's ability to adapt remains a powerful example of human resilience and capacity for change. (5)

105

How Thinking and Memory Are Affected by Vision Loss

Vision loss affects far more than just the eyes—it can influence how we think, remember, and interact with the world. Cognitive processes that depend on visual information are especially vulnerable, and adapting to this shift often requires more mental effort in daily life.

Visual Information Processing and Memory

Much of human cognition is visually driven. When eyesight is impaired, **the brain must work harder** to process incomplete or unclear visual input. This can make it more difficult to recognize faces, recall locations, or identify objects—especially in complex or unfamiliar environments. These challenges may impact working memory and recall, particularly for those who once relied heavily on visual cues to orient themselves.

Spatial Awareness and Navigation

Vision plays a key role in how we navigate through space. People with vision loss may struggle with spatial memory—remembering where things are and how to move safely through an environment. The loss of visual landmarks and depth cues requires individuals to rely more on auditory or tactile information, increasing mental effort and, in some cases, reducing confidence in mobility.

Attention and Mental Effort

With vision loss, attention must be reallocated. Tasks that once required minimal effort—like finding a seat in a room or following a moving object—now demand greater concentration and reliance on other senses. This can lead to **mental fatigue**, especially in unfamiliar or crowded settings, where constant adaptation is needed.

Social Cognition and Interaction

Visual cues are essential in human communication. Facial expressions, body language, and eye contact all provide context that helps us interpret intent and emotion. Vision loss may limit access to this information, making social interactions more mentally taxing and, at times, more awkward or confusing. This

106

can contribute to social withdrawal—not simply due to isolation, but because interactions require more effort and carry greater risk of misinterpretation.

Mental Stimulation and Emotional Health

Although vision loss does not directly cause cognitive decline, it can reduce access to the kinds of activities that help maintain brain health. Reading, driving, arts and crafts, or group games may become more difficult or less enjoyable. Over time, this reduction in cognitive engagement—combined with a higher risk of depression and anxiety—may indirectly affect memory, processing speed, and the ability to manage thoughts and actions.

Risk of Cognitive Decline: What We Know So Far

Some research suggests that vision impairment may be associated with an increased risk of cognitive decline and even dementia, including Alzheimer's disease. This *does not* mean that vision loss causes these conditions, but they may share common risk factors—such as aging, vascular disease, and genetics. Furthermore, the reduced engagement in mentally stimulating and social activities, along with the added mental strain of navigating the world with impaired sight, could contribute *indirectly* to cognitive deterioration over time. (6)

Note:

It's important to emphasize that many people with vision loss maintain strong cognitive abilities. However, recognizing the **added mental effort** involved in daily life helps families, caregivers, and professionals better support the needs of individuals with low vision. Providing accessible environments, cognitive enrichment opportunities, and emotional support can all contribute to preserving mental sharpness and quality of life.

Timing Matters: How the Age of Vision Loss Shapes Cognitive Outcomes

The age at which vision loss occurs plays a key role in how it affects memory, learning, and overall cognitive development. Vision loss early in life presents different neurological and functional challenges than vision loss later in adulthood or old age.

Early Childhood Vision Loss

When vision loss occurs during early childhood—a critical period for brain development—it can significantly influence the formation of visual memory and spatial understanding. Children with visual impairment may face challenges learning and retaining visual-based information, such as recognizing faces or understanding diagrams. These limitations can also affect their ability to interpret social cues and navigate their physical environment. (7)

However, the developing brain is remarkably adaptable. Through a process known as **neuroplasticity**, children with vision loss can recruit and strengthen non-visual pathways, especially those related to touch, hearing, and spatial awareness. Early intervention—such as Braille literacy, tactile graphics, orientation and mobility training, and multisensory learning—can support healthy cognitive and emotional development, even in the absence of vision. (7)

Adult-Onset Vision Loss

When vision loss occurs in adulthood, the brain has already established visual memory patterns, making the sudden absence of visual input more disruptive. Adults may experience difficulty recalling visual information, navigating familiar environments, or recognizing people and objects. Unlike children, adults may find it harder to rewire cognitive pathways to compensate for the loss. The added mental effort required to use alternative senses for tasks previously handled visually can increase mental fatigue and reduce efficiency in learning and daily functioning. (8)

Vision Loss and Aging

In older adults, vision loss may coincide with natural age-related cognitive changes. While **vision impairment itself does not cause dementia**, studies have shown that older individuals with vision loss are at **greater risk** for cognitive decline. This may be due to shared risk factors, such as vascular disease or genetic predisposition, as well as the impact of sensory deprivation on brain stimulation. Reduced participation in social and mentally engaging activities— often a consequence of vision impairment—can accelerate memory loss- or decision-making difficulties in some individuals. (9)

In the End...

The best way to support memory and reduce the risk of cognitive decline is to keep the brain active and engaged. For individuals with vision loss, sensory stimulation—such as listening to music or audiobooks, participating in physical activities like walking or dancing, and maintaining regular social interaction—can help stimulate the mind and promote emotional well-being.

For those with usable vision, vision rehabilitation offers important tools and training. Learning to use visual aids and compensatory strategies can help maximize remaining sight and improve independence in daily life.

It's important to remember that the impact of vision loss on memory and cognition can vary widely depending on the individual and the underlying cause of the vision loss. If you or someone you care for is experiencing memory changes or cognitive difficulties, consult with a healthcare provider. There may be treatable factors involved, and early intervention can make a meaningful difference.

References

1. **Rolls ET.** Hippocampal spatial view cells for memory and navigation, and their underlying connectivity in humans. Hippocampus. 2023 May;33(5):533-572. doi: 10.1002/hipo.23467. Epub 2022 Sep 7. PMID: 36070199; PMCID: PMC10946493.

2. Khan ZU, Martín-Montañez E, Baxter MG. Visual perception and memory systems: from cortex to medial temporal lobe. Cell Mol Life Sci. 2011 May;68(10):1737-54. doi: 10.1007/s00018-011-0641-6. Epub 2011 Mar 2. PMID: 21365279; PMCID: PMC11115075.

3. Xu Q, Liu Q, Ye C. Editorial: Cognitive mechanisms of visual attention, working memory, emotion, and their interactions. Front Neurosci. 2023 Jul 26;17:1259002. doi: 10.3389/fnins.2023.1259002. PMID: 37564371; PMCID: PMC10411335.

4. Silva PR, Farias T, Cascio F, Dos Santos L, Peixoto V, Crespo E, Ayres C, Ayres M, Marinho V, Bastos VH, Ribeiro P, Velasques B, Orsini M, Fiorelli R, de Freitas MRG, Teixeira S. Neuroplasticity in visual impairments. Neurol Int. 2018 Dec 19;10(4):7326. doi: 10.4081/ni.2018.7326. PMID: 30687464; PMCID: PMC6322049

5. Merabet LB, Pascual-Leone A. Neural reorganization following sensory loss: the opportunity of change. Nat Rev Neurosci. 2010 Jan;11(1):44-52. doi: 10.1038/nrn2758. Epub 2009 Nov 25. PMID: 19935836; PMCID: PMC3898172

6. Lee MJ, Varadaraj V, Ramulu PY, Whitson HE, Deal JA, Swenor BK. Memory and Confusion Complaints in Visually Impaired Older Adults: An Understudied Aspect of Well-Being. Gerontol Geriatr Med. 2019 Jan 8;5:2333721418818944. doi: 10.1177/2333721418818944. PMID: 30671493; PMCID: PMC6328951.

7. 4. Keil S, Fielder A, Sargent J. Management of children and young people with vision impairment: diagnosis, developmental challenges and outcomes. Arch Dis Child. 2017 Jun;102(6):566-571. doi: 10.1136/archdischild-2016-311775. Epub 2016 Nov 16. PMID: 27852581

8. Nagarajan N, Assi L, Varadaraj V, Motaghi M, Sun Y, Couser E, Ehrlich JR, Whitson H, Swenor BK. Vision impairment and cognitive decline among older adults: a systematic review. BMJ Open. 2022 Jan 6;12(1):e047929. doi: 10.1136/bmjopen-2020-047929. PMID: 34992100; PMCID: PMC8739068.

9. Runk A, Jia Y, Liu A, Chang CH, Ganguli M, Snitz BE. Associations between Visual Acuity and Cognitive Decline in Older Adulthood: A 9-Year Longitudinal Study. J Int Neuropsychol Soc. 2023 Jan;29(1):1-11. doi: 10.1017/S1355617721001363. Epub 2021 Dec 10. PMID: 36630994; PMCID: PMC9834646

In my dreams, I remember what it is to see.

When I Can See Clearly

Now and then,
a dream opens —
and I can see.

The world returns in perfect focus,
soft edges, familiar colors,
the way it used to be.

Inside the dream I whisper,
"I see everything."
And I do.

I move easily through light,
through shadow,
through the grace of sight restored —
grateful, calm,
my old self once more.

Somewhere deep inside,
the memory waits —
tiny sparks in my cortex
still reaching for a signal,
still remembering
how to see.

And when I dream,
I see again.   TC

Understanding Visual Disturbances in Low Vision

Individuals with low vision may experience a range of visual disturbances that can be confusing, unsettling, or difficult to describe. These phenomena include photopsia (flashes of light), hallucinations as seen in Charles Bonnet Syndrome, double vision, visual distortions, and halos or starbursts around lights.

This chapter provides a detailed exploration of these experiences, explaining their underlying causes, how they may present, and what they might indicate. The goal is to help you better understand these symptoms and know when to seek professional advice.

1. **Photopsia**
2. **Hallucinations of Charles Bonnet Syndrome**
3. **Distortions**
4. **Double Vision**
5. **Halos and Starburst Patterns around lights**

1. Photopsia

Photopsia refers to the perception of flashes or patterns of light that appear without any actual light stimulus. These light phenomena can vary in appearance—from brief flashes to moving, flickering shapes—and may occur in one or both eyes. Importantly, photopsia in individuals with vision loss typically arises spontaneously and without any visual triggers in the environment.

This phenomenon is commonly reported by individuals with degenerative retinal diseases such as **retinitis pigmentosa**, **age-related macular degeneration (AMD)**, and **Stargardt disease**. In these conditions, photopsia is believed to result from residual neurological activity in damaged areas of the retina. One theory suggests that the abnormal firing of "sick" or dying retinal cells causes these spontaneous visual events, much like the phantom limb pain experienced by amputees. In both cases, sensory cells continue to send signals despite the absence of normal input. (1)

Other Types of Flashes Not the Result of Vision Loss

It is important to distinguish photopsia related to retinal degeneration from light flashes caused by **retinal detachment** or **retinal traction**, which are potentially sight-threatening. These flashes are due to mechanical stimulation of the retina—for example, from a retinal tear or vitreous pulling on the retina—and warrant immediate medical attention, as they can signal the beginning of a retinal detachment or the formation of a retinal hole.

Phosphenes

Phosphenes are another phenomenon involving flashes or bursts of light, but they are typically harmless. They occur when the retina is mechanically stimulated from outside the eye—such as by rubbing the eyes, sneezing, or experiencing a blow to the head. This produces the common sensation of "seeing stars." Unlike photopsia in retinal disease, phosphenes are transient, situational, and usually benign.

Ocular Migraine Aura

(*Also known as retinal, visual, or eye migraines*)

Ocular migraines may affect individuals with normal vision as well as those with vision impairment. They present as temporary visual disturbances with distinct features:

- Area of blocked, grey or white vision with scintillating 'broken shards of glass' flashing lights,
- starts small in an area and seems to expand until finally dissipating,
- lasts from 5 to 20 minutes,
- usually in one eye, but often can't tell if it is one or both eyes,
- may happen multiple times in one day.

The exact cause of ocular migraines remains uncertain, but the most widely accepted explanation involves **vasospasm of the retinal blood vessels**. This temporary reduction in retinal blood flow is thought to produce the light phenomena and transient vision loss. While ocular migraines are generally considered harmless and without lasting effects, frequent or new-onset episodes should prompt a medical evaluation to rule out other causes.

2. Vision Loss, Hallucinations, and Charles Bonnet Syndrome

Charles Bonnet Syndrome (CBS) refers to visual hallucinations experienced by individuals with significant vision loss. It is commonly, but mistakenly, assumed to affect only elderly people with low vision. While CBS is indeed more frequently reported in older adults, documented cases have also occurred in children with visual impairment.

A major challenge in identifying CBS lies in underreporting. Many individuals—both young and old—are reluctant to disclose visual hallucinations for fear of being misunderstood, labeled as cognitively impaired, or considered mentally ill. This stigma can delay or prevent appropriate diagnosis and support.

Common Traits Among Those Who Experience CBS

Those most likely to experience CBS are individuals who:

- Have recently lost vision, although CBS can occur in those with long-standing vision loss as well,
- Have bilateral vision loss (typically 20/100 or worse in both eyes), and
- Are cognitively intact, mentally alert, and aware that the hallucinations are not real.

Triggers and Causes

CBS hallucinations are more likely to occur under specific conditions, such as:

- Living alone or experiencing social isolation,
- Being in quiet, dimly lit environments (such as lying in bed at night),
- Periods of fatigue, stress, or sensory deprivation.

The condition is most often associated with age-related eye diseases, particularly **age-related macular degeneration (AMD)**. However, it can also occur in individuals with **cataracts**, **glaucoma**, **diabetic retinopathy**, **optic neuropathy**, **retinitis pigmentosa**, or any disorder that causes significant visual disruption along the visual pathway, including within the brain.

Charles Bonnet Syndrome in Children

Though CBS is predominantly observed in adults, there are confirmed reports of the syndrome in children. Pediatric cases, while less common, offer valuable insights into the broad spectrum of individuals who may experience CBS.

A study published in the *British Journal of Ophthalmology* examined CBS in children with visual impairment and found that children as young as five years old can experience visual hallucinations. These ranged from simple patterns or shapes to complex and vivid scenes involving animals or people. (2)

This study emphasized the need for increased awareness of CBS among healthcare providers, educators, and caregivers. Diagnosing CBS in children can be particularly difficult, as young patients may struggle to describe their experiences clearly, and adults may misinterpret their reports as imagination or fantasy.

Additional case reports and anecdotal evidence support the occurrence of CBS in children with retinal dystrophies or congenital blindness. These accounts highlight the importance of listening to children's descriptions of visual phenomena and recognizing the possibility of CBS—even at a young age.

'Phantom Vision'

The visual hallucinations experienced in Charles Bonnet Syndrome (CBS) are believed to result from sudden or significant vision loss due to damage anywhere along the visual system—whether in the eyes, neural pathways, or the occipital cortex at the back of the brain.

These hallucinations are often compared to the *phantom pain* experienced by amputees—where the brain continues to perceive sensations, including pain, from a missing limb. In the case of vision loss, the brain, deprived of normal visual input, "fills in the blanks" with internally generated imagery. While the eye itself does not feel pain, it can experience *phantom vision* in the form of spontaneous, vivid hallucinations. These phantom visions are the hallmark of Charles Bonnet Syndrome.

What Do People See?

The hallucinations associated with CBS range from simple patterns or geometric lines to elaborate scenes involving people, animals, or fantastical landscapes. They may appear cartoon-like, unusually small or distorted, and sometimes grotesque. Despite their surreal nature, the images are often reported to be brilliantly detailed and seamlessly blended into the environment.

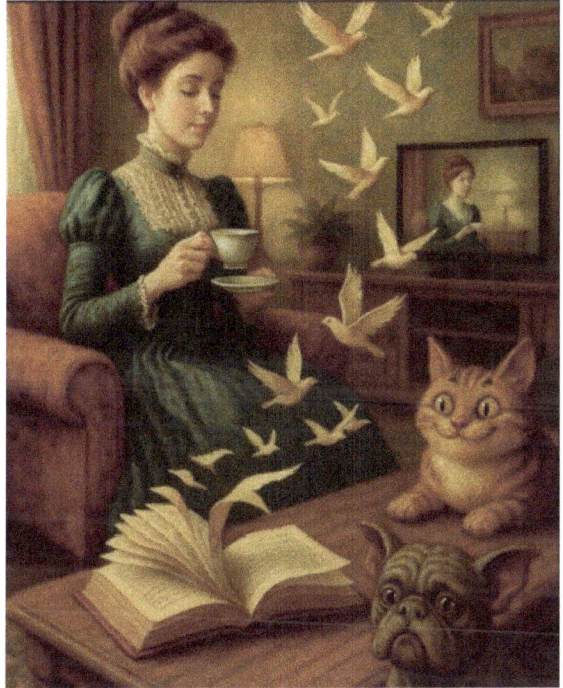

These episodes can be fleeting—lasting only seconds—or persist for hours. Importantly, the hallucinations **do not interact** with the person experiencing them. Individuals describe themselves as passive observers rather than active participants. Though some may find these visions unsettling or intrusive, they are typically *not* described as frightening or threatening.

Realistic but fantastic. AI-generated illustration created using OpenAI tools.

Managing Charles Bonnet Syndrome

Some people find the hallucinations distressing enough to seek medical help, especially if unaware that CBS is a known condition. Currently, there is no specific treatment to eliminate the hallucinations directly. In cases where vision loss is reversible—such as cataracts—surgical correction may reduce or resolve the hallucinations. However, in most cases, vision cannot be restored.

There are coping strategies that may help dispel or shorten the hallucinations when they occur. These include:

- Changing lighting conditions
- Blinking rapidly or closing the eyes
- Shifting eye position or moving the head
- Engaging in stimulating activities to re-direct visual attention

Reducing social isolation and participating in vision rehabilitation programs can also be beneficial. The use of optical aids or assistive technology may help re-engage the visual system and minimize the occurrence or intensity of phantom visions.

3. Distortion of Vision

People often report that images, lines, or print appear curved or warped when wearing a new pair of glasses. This type of distortion typically disappears once the glasses are removed and is a common experience—even among individuals with normal vision—who may be sensitive to changes in their prescription.

For individuals with low vision, distortion may also occur when using magnifying devices. The optics of some low vision aids can create visual distortion, especially along the edges of the lens. In such cases, switching to a different type or strength of magnifier often resolves the problem.

Distortion Associated with Eye Disease

In contrast to optical distortion from glasses or magnifiers, visual distortion caused by eye disease is typically persistent and directly related to the underlying pathology responsible for the vision loss. These distortions do not resolve by removing glasses or changing magnifiers.

Clear, sharp images depend on the retina being smooth and properly aligned against the back wall of the eye. When the retina is raised, wrinkled, or displaced, the image it sends to the brain is similarly altered—resulting in distortion.

Examples of disease-related causes of distortion include:

- **Fluid accumulation beneath the retina** – such as in *wet age-related macular degeneration*, where leaking blood vessels elevate portions of the retina.
- **Disruption of photoreceptor cell alignment** – often due to *drusen deposits*, which crowd and shift retinal cells out of position.
- **Retinal contraction or wrinkling** – caused by *epiretinal membranes* (scar tissue), which can pull on the retina and make images appear smaller, crowded, or misshapen.

Sometimes these changes are subtle, and while not always treatable, they are important to monitor closely to detect progression.

A common tool used to monitor central visual distortion in those with retinal disease is the **Amsler Grid**.

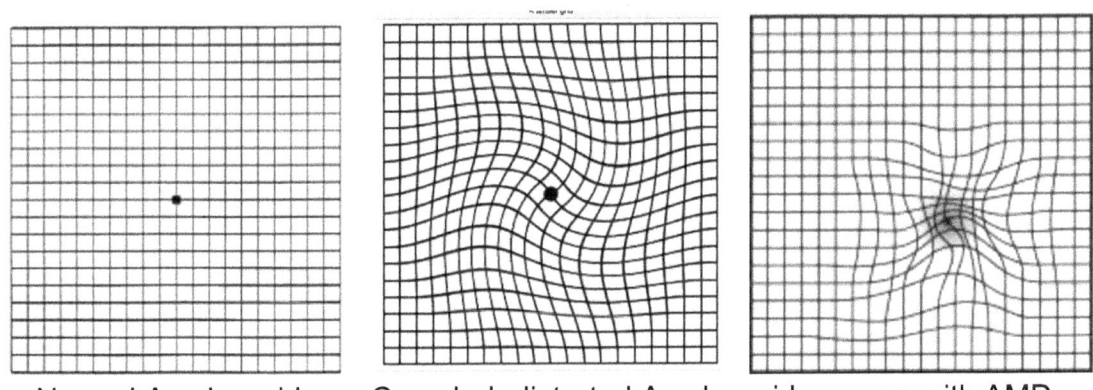

Normal Amsler grid   Crowded, distorted Amsler grid as seen with AMD

The Amsler Grid consists of a pattern of straight horizontal and vertical lines printed on a square sheet. To use it, the individual covers one eye and holds the grid approximately 11 inches (28–30 cm) from the open eye. While staring directly at the central dot, they are asked to notice whether any lines appear wavy, missing, blurred, or distorted. These observations can signal subtle changes in the macula or central retina and should be reported to an eye care provider promptly.

4. Double vision (also known as Diplopia)

Double vision, or *diplopia*, is the perception of seeing two images of a single object. It is generally categorized into two types:

- **Monocular double vision:** Persists when only one eye is open.
- **Binocular double vision:** Occurs only when both eyes are open and disappears when one eye is closed.

In individuals with normal vision, both eyes are aligned and work together to create a single, unified image. This binocular coordination is essential for accurate depth perception, sharp visual acuity, balance, and coordinated movement.

Causes of Binocular Double Vision

Binocular diplopia typically results from a misalignment of the eyes, which can be caused by a variety of conditions, including:

- **Eye muscle dysfunction:** Often due to inflammation (such as in thyroid eye disease), nerve palsy, or trauma to the orbit.
- **Vascular conditions:** Including stroke, aneurysm, or diabetic microvascular complications.
- **Neurological disorders:** Such as multiple sclerosis, myasthenia gravis, or brain lesions affecting cranial nerves.
- **Decompensated phoria:** In individuals with minor, latent misalignments (phorias), the brain and eye muscles usually maintain single vision. However, those with vision loss may struggle to compensate for the misalignment, resulting in double vision. (3)

Causes of Monocular Double Vision

Monocular diplopia persists when viewing with just one eye and often arises from structural issues within the eye itself. Common causes include:

1. **Astigmatism:**
   An irregular curvature of the cornea that can cause ghosting or doubling of images. This is common in both normally sighted and low vision individuals and is typically correctable with glasses or contact lenses.

2. **Corneal Disease:**
   Any disruption of the smooth, refractive surface of the cornea can cause light to scatter and produce double or distorted images. Causes include:
   - **Scarring** from trauma or past infections
   - **Corneal swelling (edema):** Resulting from trauma, infections, or certain eye surgeries
   - **Keratoconus:** A progressive thinning and weakening of the cornea, which causes it to bulge into a cone shape. This deformation can lead to both image distortion and monocular diplopia.

3. **Lens Abnormalities:**
   Disturbances in the lens of the eye can also result in monocular double vision:
   - **Cataracts:** Clouding or structural changes in the lens (e.g., vacuoles or fluid clefts) can cause light to scatter, producing ghosted or double images.
   - **Dislocated intraocular lens (IOL):** In individuals who have had cataract surgery, trauma can cause the implanted artificial lens to shift from its intended position, resulting in monocular double vision.

4. **Retinal Disease:**
   Swelling or structural disruption of the retina, particularly in the macula, can displace photoreceptor alignment and lead to visual disturbances such as blurring, distortion, and sometimes ghosting or doubling of images. Conditions that may cause retinal swelling include:
   - **Wet macular degeneration**
   - **Diabetic retinopathy**
   - **Uveitis**
   - **Inflammatory diseases:** Such as viral retinitis or toxoplasmosis
   - **Autoimmune diseases:** Including sarcoidosis, Behçet's Syndrome, and Vogt-Koyanagi-Harada disease

Understanding the type and cause of double vision is important for effective treatment and management. While some forms of diplopia may resolve with corrective lenses, prisms, or surgery, others may signal underlying neurological or muscular issues that require further investigation. For individuals with low vision, the experience of double vision can compound existing visual challenges, making daily activities even more difficult. By recognizing the signs and seeking appropriate care, individuals and caregivers can better navigate this often-disorienting symptom and reduce its impact on quality of life.

5. Halos and Starburst Patterns

Halos and starbursts are visual phenomena in which bright lights appear to be surrounded by glowing rings or radiate streaks outward like a star. While these effects may seem merely decorative, they can severely impair night vision, depth perception, and overall visual clarity—especially in low-light environments such as driving.

These disturbances are usually symptoms of underlying eye conditions that affect how light enters and travels through the eye, particularly involving the **cornea**, **lens**, or intraocular structures. Understanding their causes helps individuals seek appropriate treatment and manage their visual challenges more effectively.

Common Causes:

1. Cataracts

Cataracts are the most frequent cause of halos and starbursts, especially in older adults. Alongside blurred or dimmed vision and increased light sensitivity, patients may notice prominent glare and radiating light patterns—most commonly at night.

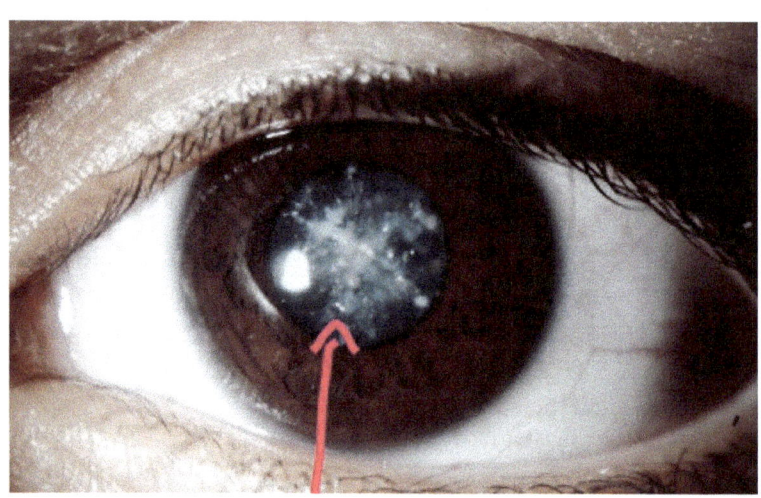

Senile cortical cataracts

These effects result from structural changes in the crystalline lens, where the formation of vacuoles, clefts, splits, or granulations scatters incoming light. This scattering creates the distinctive halo or starburst effect around light sources.

2. Intraocular Lens Implants (IOLs)

After cataract surgery, the natural lens is replaced with an artificial intraocular lens (IOL). In some individuals, particularly in the early post-operative period, the IOL may cause **dysphotopsia**—unwanted optical side effects due to reflections off the lens or its edge. These may appear as glare, starbursts, halos, or even dark shadows in peripheral vision.

3. Corneal Edema (Swelling)

The cornea, made up of multiple cell layers, plays an important role in focusing light. If disrupted by disease, injury, or surgery, the cornea can accumulate fluid and become swollen, leading to light scatter and visual distortion. Halos, cloudiness, and glare are common symptoms.

Conditions associated with corneal edema include:

- Fuchs' corneal dystrophy
- Acute angle-closure glaucoma
- Keratoconus
- Postoperative corneal swelling (e.g., after cataract surgery)

Halos and starbursts are not just minor nuisances—they can significantly affect functional vision, especially in low-light conditions. Recognizing these patterns and understanding their potential causes can guide individuals toward appropriate interventions or evaluations. While they may sometimes be managed with optical or medical strategies, persistent symptoms should prompt further investigation by an eye care professional.

In the End...

Although individuals with normal vision may occasionally experience unusual visual phenomena, certain disturbances are particularly characteristic of eye disease. Some of these serve as early warning signs of an underlying condition, while others are direct consequences of the disease process itself.

While a number of visual disturbances can be treated or managed, many remain persistent and challenging for those with low vision. Gaining an understanding of these effects is essential—not only for those living with visual impairment but also for their families and caregivers. This awareness can foster more effective support, guide medical attention, and help individuals adapt to the visual challenges they face.

References:

1. Borruat FX. Photopsia: an often unrecognized symptom and sensitivity of electroretinography]. Klin Monbl Augenheilkd. 1998 May;212(5):394-6. French. doi: 10.1055/s-2008-1034916. PMID: 9677589.

2. Jones L, Moosajee M. Visual hallucinations and sight loss in children and young adults: a retrospective case series of Charles Bonnet syndrome. Br J Ophthalmol. 2021 Nov;105(11):1604-1609. doi: 10.1136/bjophthalmol-2020-317237. Epub 2020 Sep 15. PMID: 32933935; PMCID: PMC8543192.

3. Ali MH, Berry S, Qureshi A, Rattanalert N, Demer JL. Decompensated Esophoria as a Benign Cause of Acquired Esotropia. Am J Ophthalmol. 2018 Oct;194:95-100. doi: 10.1016/j.ajo.2018.07.007. Epub 2018 Jul 24. PMID: 30053478; PMCID: PMC6438619.

Understanding Why Those with Vision Loss Have a Problem with Facial Recognition

Recognizing faces is a fundamental part of human interaction, essential for social connection, communication, and emotional recognition. However, individuals with low vision—particularly those with central vision loss—often struggle with this task.

Accurate facial recognition depends on the ability to perceive fine detail and maintain steady focus, both of which are compromised in many low vision conditions. Common causes of facial recognition difficulty include macular degeneration, Stargardt disease, and various inherited cone-rod dystrophies, all of which affect the central retina responsible for processing detailed visual information.

Two Factors Contributing to Decreased Facial Recognition Ability

1. Reduced Visual Acuity

Facial recognition depends heavily on the ability to perceive fine details—such as the shape and spacing of the eyes, nose, and mouth. However, individuals with low vision often experience significant reductions in visual acuity, especially when the macula, the part of the retina responsible for sharp central vision, is damaged. When visual input from this area is blurred or distorted, the brain receives an incomplete or unstable image, making it difficult to identify and remember unique facial features. (1)

Even when individuals attempt to rely on a peripheral area of the retina for visual input, this region lacks the dense concentration of cone photoreceptors found in the macula. As a result, it cannot support the same level of detail discrimination. This makes it harder to perceive subtle facial differences that are essential for recognition.

To compensate, individuals with low vision may focus on more general or easily observed characteristics, such as face shape, hairstyle, posture, or voice. While they might be able to identify the presence of facial features—eyes, nose, mouth—the finer distinguishing details remain blurred or indiscernible.

2. Eccentric Viewing and Unstable Fixation

In more advanced cases of central vision loss, individuals often adapt by using a technique known as *eccentric viewing*. This involves training themselves to use a healthier, functioning region of the retina outside the damaged macula to view objects. (2) This alternative area, often referred to as the preferred retinal locus (PRL), becomes the new focal point for gathering visual information.

However, this adaptive strategy has its limitations. The PRL and surrounding peripheral retinal areas are not optimized for fixation stability or detail resolution. The retinal wiring and reduced cone density in these areas make it more difficult to "lock onto" a target—such as a face—and hold a steady gaze. In contrast, the central vision area (when intact) can maintain stable fixation, allowing the brain to efficiently analyze facial details and link them to memory.

Because the peripheral retina does not process visual input as precisely, facial recognition becomes even more compromised. Despite their efforts to "push aside" the central blind spot, individuals using eccentric viewing still struggle to interpret and retain accurate images of faces.

The Challenge of Facial Expression Interpretation for the Visually Impaired

The Importance of Facial Expressions in Communication

Facial expressions are a powerful form of nonverbal communication, conveying emotions, reactions, and social cues that enhance spoken language. These expressions are interpreted rapidly and unconsciously, enabling individuals to recognize a wide range of emotions and personality traits that may not be conveyed through tone of voice or words alone.

Emotions such as happiness, sadness, anger, fear, surprise, or even subtle cues like skepticism or distraction are communicated through facial movements. These visual signals enrich conversations, helping listeners grasp the speaker's emotional state and intentions more fully. In typical face-to-face interactions, people often respond by mirroring each other's expressions, fostering empathy and connection.

However, individuals with visual impairment are deprived of this essential layer of communication. Without access to facial cues, they may struggle to interpret the emotional context of a conversation. This limitation can result in misunderstandings, where the visually impaired person might seem indifferent or unresponsive—not because they lack empathy, but because they lack the visual input to guide their reactions.

Instead, they must rely heavily on verbal indicators such as tone, pitch, and volume. While these cues can convey emotion to some extent, they often lack the nuance provided by facial expressions. As a result, social interactions may become stressful or confusing, leading to feelings of discomfort, anxiety, or even embarrassment.

Over time, some individuals with low vision may begin to withdraw from social settings, not due to disinterest, but because of the difficulty and frustration of navigating conversations without the benefit of visual emotional cues—an integral part of human connection.

Social Embarrassment

Recognizing a face offers more than emotional expression; it conveys age, gender, familiarity, and focus of attention. When a person with low vision cannot correctly identify to whom a comment or question is directed—or mistakenly greets someone—they may unintentionally embarrass themselves. Misidentifications or conversational misfires can be unsettling for both the visually impaired individual and the people around them.

Social Awkwardness

Eye contact plays a central role in building trust and connection during conversation. Those unable to see well enough to make eye contact may be perceived as evasive, uninterested, or overly shy. These misinterpretations can strain both personal and professional relationships, further complicating communication.

Social Anxiety

Repeated experiences of embarrassment or misunderstanding can lead to growing self-consciousness and anxiety. The visually impaired person may dread social encounters, particularly in group settings, where identifying voices or tracking conversations becomes more difficult. Fear of making mistakes may cause them to withdraw socially.

Social Isolation

Over time, the challenges of reading faces, maintaining eye contact, and confidently engaging in conversation may cause individuals with vision loss to avoid social settings altogether. The inability to respond naturally to nonverbal cues or facial expressions can make them feel emotionally disconnected — alone, even in the company of others.

The Case for Emojis

Think about reading a text message and being unsure of the writer's intent. Are they angry, joking, sarcastic, or annoyed? Without facial expression or tone of voice, it's hard to tell. This is the same kind of uncertainty people with visual impairment often experience in face-to-face conversations. They may miss subtle cues like a smirk, a wink, or a raised eyebrow—nonverbal signals that provide context and meaning.

Fortunately, in written communication, we can use emojis to fill in those emotional blanks. But in real life, there's no emoji to help clarify someone's facial expression. That's the social gap many visually impaired individuals must learn to navigate.

The Challenge of Enjoying Movies and Television for the Visually Impaired

For individuals with visual impairment, watching movies or television presents unique challenges. One of the most significant is the inability to clearly interpret facial expressions—an essential aspect of understanding characters' emotions and intentions. Without this visual feedback, viewers may struggle to follow the storyline or emotionally connect with the characters.

In addition to facial expressions, visual media often relies heavily on nonverbal storytelling elements such as body language, subtle gestures, setting details, and scene transitions. These cues help convey mood, plot developments, and relationships between characters, but they can be difficult or impossible to perceive with low vision.

Audio descriptions—narrated explanations of visual elements inserted during natural pauses in dialogue—offer an important accessibility solution. They allow visually impaired viewers to follow the visual context more fully. Unfortunately, not all films or television programs include audio description tracks, especially older content or programs on less accessible platforms.

Without these supports, watching a movie or television show can become a frustrating experience, as visually impaired viewers may miss critical narrative elements that sighted audiences often take for granted.

Making Connections Without Sight: Adaptive Strategies

For individuals with low vision, recognizing faces can be challenging. However, there are several techniques that can help compensate for this difficulty and make social interactions more comfortable and successful:

1. Use Voice Recognition
A friendly "Hello" and a smile can prompt the other person to speak, allowing you to identify them by their voice. Voice is often a reliable cue, especially for people you know well.

2. Get Closer
Decreasing the distance between yourself and the person you are interacting with, is a form of magnification. A closer distance makes the identifying features easier to interpret. *Fair warning:* getting so close as to enter into someone's personal space can make them uncomfortable and make the interaction feel awkward.

129

3. Rely on General Physical Clues
When facial details are unclear, broader characteristics can help—such as height, build, posture, hairstyle, or the shape of the head. These clues are especially useful for recognizing familiar individuals you see regularly.

4. Practice Short-Term Memorization
Remembering what someone is wearing, including the color and style of clothing or their hairstyle, can help you identify them during a single visit. You can also associate people with consistent patterns, such as where they usually sit, their job role, or unique speech habits or mannerisms.

5. A Willing Partner, Friend, or Assistant.
If the person who often accompanies you understands the dilemma of not being able to instantly recognize someone, a well-versed companion can be an asset by whispering an identifying name. Not always available, but helpful when they are around

Do Those with Vision Loss and Problems with Facial Recognition have Prosopagnosia?

Prosopagnosia, also known as face blindness or facial agnosia, is a neurological condition that affects a person's ability to recognize faces. Unlike vision impairment or memory loss, prosopagnosia is caused by damage or developmental abnormalities in a specific region of the brain known as the **right fusiform gyrus**. This area plays a key role in processing facial features and linking them to stored memories.

Because prosopagnosia results from a **brain-based dysfunction**, individuals with visual impairment who struggle to recognize faces **do not** have prosopagnosia. Their difficulty stems from degraded visual input, not from an inability of the brain to process facial identity

Facial Recognition Technology for the Visually Impaired

What if, instead of relying on a companion or friend to help recognize faces, an artificial intelligence system could whisper identities and emotions into your ear?

Facial recognition technology is rapidly evolving, and developers are working to adapt it for people with visual impairments. These tools aim to serve as real-time digital assistants—an "extra set of eyes" capable of identifying individuals and interpreting their facial expressions in a variety of environments.

One of the main challenges in developing such systems is the complexity of facial recognition itself. Algorithms must handle wide variations in lighting, facial angles, and expressions. They must also ensure privacy, manage large databases securely, and work seamlessly in real-world settings, not just controlled environments. (3)

Several promising approaches are under active development:

- **Wearable AI Devices:** Smart glasses and headsets equipped with cameras, facial recognition software, and bone-conduction or in-ear audio are being tested. These devices can scan faces in real time and compare them with a stored database of known individuals, announcing the identity and emotional expression to the user. For example, OrCam MyEye and Envision Glasses already provide some object and face recognition capabilities, although expression reading is still in its early stages. (4, 5)
- **Smart Canes:** Researchers have proposed smart canes integrated with computer vision systems capable of detecting and identifying faces. While most current smart cane prototypes focus on obstacle detection, the incorporation of facial recognition is a logical next step, combining mobility and social accessibility in a single device. (5)
- **Mobile Apps:** Smartphone apps are being developed to assist with facial recognition in both physical and digital spaces. Some experimental apps can describe facial expressions in images from social media platforms or text message attachments, helping the user interpret visual content that others take for granted. For example, apps like **Seeing AI by Microsoft** include basic facial recognition features and can describe a person's age, gender, and emotional expression. (5)

A notable setback occurred when Facebook shut down its automated facial recognition system in November 2021, citing privacy concerns. However, smaller-scale, opt-in technologies continue to evolve, emphasizing user control,

131

secure data storage, and personalized databases to respect individual privacy. (6)

While we are not yet at the point of seamless, real-time facial recognition integrated into daily life for the visually impaired, the foundation has been laid. With advances in AI, wearables, and edge computing, this type of assistance is no longer science fiction—it's on the near horizon.

In the End:

The ability to recognize faces plays an important role in personal, social, and professional relationships. People with low vision often experience social embarrassment, anxiety, and fear due to this challenge. Their communication can be hindered by difficulty in reading facial expressions, which are key to understanding emotions and intentions. Although many develop strategies to navigate social situations, persistent fears and reduced confidence can lead to increased anxiety and avoidance of social interactions.

References

1. Seiple W, Rosen RB, Garcia PM. Abnormal fixation in individuals with age-related macular degeneration when viewing an image of a face. Optom Vis Sci. 2013 Jan;90(1):45-56. doi: 10.1097/OPX.0b013e3182794775. PMID: 23238260.

2. Seiple W, Rosen RB, Garcia PM. Abnormal fixation in individuals with age-related macular degeneration when viewing an image of a face. Optom Vis Sci. 2013 Jan;90(1):45-56. doi: 10.1097/OPX.0b013e3182794775. PMID: 23238260.

3. Robust Face Recognition Under Challenging Conditions: A Comprehensive Review of Deep Learning Methods and Challenges. (2025). *Applied Sciences, 15*(17), 9390. https://doi.org/10.3390/app15179390

4. Seiple, W., van der Aa, H. P. A., Garcia-Piña, F., Greco, I., Roberts, C., & van Nispen, R. (2025). Performance on Activities of Daily Living and User Experience When Using Artificial Intelligence by Individuals With Vision mpairment. *Translational Vision Science & Technology, 14*(1), 3.

5. Naayini, P., Myakala, P. K., Bura, C., Jonnalagadda, A. K., & Kamatala, S. (2025). AI-Powered Assistive Technologies for Visual Impairment. *arXiv*.

6. American Library Association. (2021) Facebook and the Biometric Information Privacy Act Litigation. Endnotes, 11(1).

Understanding Loneliness and Social Isolation

Loneliness and social isolation can arise from many interconnected factors and can significantly diminish quality of life for individuals living with vision loss. Although these terms are often used interchangeably, they represent distinct experiences and affect individuals in different ways.

Loneliness refers to a subjective, psychosocial sense of emotional disconnection from others. It is the painful feeling that meaningful social or personal connections are missing, even when people are physically present. **Social isolation**, by contrast, describes an objective lack of social contact, relationships, or opportunities for engagement. Isolation may be self-imposed, or it may result from limited access to transportation, support services, or inclusive environments. A person who is socially isolated may not necessarily feel lonely and may even prefer minimal interaction, while someone who is frequently surrounded by others may still experience profound loneliness.

Social support plays an important role in protecting against both loneliness and social isolation. Social support consists of relationships with family, friends, and others who provide emotional understanding, companionship, and practical assistance. Importantly, it is the quality—not merely the number—of these relationships that matters most. Individuals who have supportive, respectful, and nonjudgmental relationships are better equipped to cope with vision loss and are less likely to withdraw or feel alone. In contrast, those who lack reliable, understanding connections are at greater risk for isolation and the emotional distress that often accompanies it.

Factors That Contribute to Loneliness and Social Isolation in Vision Loss

1. Reduced Opportunities for Social Engagement

Employment provides more than financial stability—it offers daily social interaction, purpose, and a sense of belonging. Individuals with vision loss who are unemployed or underemployed often lose access to these built-in social connections. Employers or coworkers may incorrectly assume that a person with vision loss can no longer perform their job, even when reasonable accommodations would allow them to continue working effectively.

Physical activity and sports are also important contributors to both physical and mental well-being. However, individuals with visual impairments are frequently excluded from these activities due to concerns about safety or misconceptions about ability. This exclusion is particularly harmful for children, for whom participation in sports and group activities plays an important role in social development and peer connection. (1)

2. Loss of Emotional Cues in Social Interaction

Social interaction relies heavily on visual and emotional cues such as facial expressions, body language, and eye contact. When these cues are missed or misinterpreted, face-to-face interactions may feel incomplete, awkward, or frustrating. Individuals with vision loss may worry about appearing aloof, unintelligent, awkward, or socially disengaged, even when they are fully invested in the interaction.

Vision loss can also lead to subtle but painful social experiences, such as being ignored or spoken around. Family members, healthcare providers, or others may direct questions to a spouse, caregiver, or companion instead of speaking directly to the person with vision loss. These experiences contribute to emotional loneliness—being physically present yet feeling unseen, misunderstood, or excluded.

Over time, repeated awkward or dismissive interactions can make social situations feel unsafe. To protect themselves emotionally, individuals may withdraw or avoid these settings altogether, increasing the risk of loneliness and isolation.

3. Barriers to Visual Cues in the Environment

Difficulties with facial recognition, seeing gestures such as a wave across the room, or interpreting visual details in the environment can reduce situational awareness and confidence in social settings. Poor lighting, excessive background noise, and visually complex public spaces further interfere with effective communication and connection. (2)

In public environments, impatience from others—eye rolls, sighs, or visible frustration when extra time is needed to read a menu, sign a receipt, or navigate a checkout line—can be deeply discouraging. As a result, individuals with vision loss may begin to avoid crowded or unfamiliar environments, favoring one-to-one interactions where they feel more comfortable and in control. Over time, this avoidance can limit participation in clubs, events, and community organizations. (3)

4. Limited Mobility and Resources

Transportation is one of the most significant barriers to social participation for individuals with vision loss, particularly for those living in rural areas. Without reliable transportation, opportunities to attend social events, appointments, or community activities are sharply reduced.

Older adults with vision loss are especially vulnerable, as they may have fewer family members or friends available to assist with transportation. Lack of transportation directly inhibits social inclusion. Individuals with vision impairment are less likely to leave their homes when transportation options are limited, a problem that disproportionately affects older adults. (4)

Concerns about personal safety also play a role. Navigating sidewalks, crossing streets with moving traffic, or finding one's way through unfamiliar public buildings can feel overwhelming. For many older adults, frustration with decreased mobility and the need for assisted guidance may further discourage independent outings, contributing to isolation.

5. Anxiety and Depression

Vision loss is a well-established risk factor for both depression and anxiety. While these conditions may initially arise from fears related to disease progression, uncertainty about the future, or changes in independence, social withdrawal can intensify symptoms. Loneliness and isolation do not merely coexist with depression and anxiety—they often exacerbate them.

In social situations where communication is difficult or patience is lacking, individuals with vision loss may feel ignored or excluded. Repeated experiences of misunderstanding or marginalization can increase emotional distress, leading individuals to retreat into what feels like a safer, more controlled emotional space. Unfortunately, this withdrawal often deepens both loneliness and psychological distress.

6. Difficulty Performing Activities of Daily Living

Vision loss can bring an emotional burden as individuals experience changes in their ability to perform activities of daily living such as reading mail, cooking, managing medications, or moving freely without assistance. These challenges can negatively affect self-perception, leading individuals to feel diminished or "less than" others. Embarrassment about needing help may further discourage social engagement.

Well-intended but unsolicited assistance can compound this effect. Others may grab an arm without asking, take over tasks, or insist on helping even when the individual is capable of managing independently. When individuals lose confidence in completing daily tasks, they may feel a growing sense of dependence and loss of control.

In an effort to regain control, some individuals pull back from helpers or deny themselves assistance, choosing to do without rather than feel dependent. While understandable, this response can inadvertently increase isolation. (5)

7. Individual Factors

Not everyone with vision loss experiences loneliness in the same way. Individual factors such as age, motivation, resilience, attitudes to life, self-esteem, personal history, cultural background, and social expectations all influence how someone adjusts.

Older adults may be less motivated to learn new skills or adopt assistive technologies, increasing the likelihood of reduced activity and social engagement. In contrast, individuals with higher self-esteem and confidence in their abilities are more likely to attempt problem-solving, seek support, and remain socially engaged.

Negative past experiences, repeated failures, or limited access to resources can erode confidence. When individuals lose trust in their own abilities, they may withdraw socially and underestimate their capacity to adapt.

8. Socioeconomic Factors

Socioeconomic status plays a significant role in loneliness and social isolation among individuals with vision loss. Studies show a strong association between visual impairment, reduced income security, and social isolation. (2) Individuals with limited financial resources face additional barriers, including higher medical costs, insurance challenges, transportation expenses, the need for assistive services, and the cost of visual aids and accommodations.

Those at lower income levels are at greater risk for loneliness and isolation, as financial strain limits access to both social opportunities and supportive resources.

9. Social Stigma and Discrimination

Social stigmatization is a pervasive and often overlooked aspect of vision loss. It refers to the negative attitudes, assumptions, or judgments directed toward individuals with visual impairment, resulting in being treated differently rather than seen as whole, capable people. Stigma may present as pity, impatience, avoidance, or assumptions about intelligence or competence.

People may speak louder, slower, or more simply, mistakenly believing that vision loss also affects hearing or cognitive ability. Social expectations and misconceptions—shaped by a society designed for the sighted—can result in discrimination in employment, housing, healthcare, and even personal relationships. These attitudes quietly push individuals with vision loss to the margins, fostering exclusion and isolation.

Stigma affects not only how others behave, but also how individuals begin to view themselves. Repeated experiences of misunderstanding or judgment may lead individuals to withdraw socially to protect themselves. (5) Activities that were once enjoyable—dining out, attending events, traveling, or running errands—can begin to feel stressful or embarrassing.

Some individuals avoid using visual aids such as white canes, magnifiers, or electronic devices in public due to fear of being stared at, pitied, or labeled as "disabled." (5, 6)

Research shows that discrimination associated with vision loss is not merely a subjective perception. Population-based studies from England and the United States demonstrate that individuals with visual impairment report higher rates of everyday discrimination than those with typical vision. These experiences are associated with increased depression, loneliness, and reduced quality of life and life satisfaction. (7)

Discrimination occurs across multiple settings—from public spaces to healthcare environments—and affects daily life in profound ways. Over time, avoidance of social situations may feel protective, but it reinforces a cycle in which withdrawal leads to loneliness, and loneliness deepens social isolation. Someone may be physically present among others, yet feel profoundly alone.

Supporting Social Development in Children with Vision Loss

Research shows that children and adolescents with vision loss tend to have smaller social circles than their sighted peers and are at greater risk for social isolation. (2) Sighted children typically have more opportunities to participate in organized social activities such as sports, clubs, and group recreation. In contrast, children with visual impairments are often excluded from these activities due to the visual demands involved and concerns about safety, even when participation could be possible with appropriate adaptations.

These barriers can significantly contribute to social isolation. Children and adolescents with vision loss may also be less likely to initiate social interactions, particularly in unfamiliar settings. (2) During childhood and adolescence—periods marked by heightened self-consciousness—concerns about appearing different or being judged by peers can further discourage social engagement.

Developing social skills early in life is critical to reducing the risk of loneliness and isolation. However, this process is often more challenging for children with vision loss due to limited access to visual and emotional cues such as facial expressions, gestures, and group dynamics. These limitations can affect the development of independence and interpersonal relationships. Additionally, children with visual impairments may be more vulnerable to bullying, teasing, or ridicule, further reinforcing withdrawal.

Children may also struggle to explain their visual limitations to peers. When others do not understand why a child behaves differently—such as standing closer, missing visual cues, or avoiding certain activities—misunderstandings can arise, leading to exclusion and stigmatization.

Children who are supported in making adjustments and adaptations at an early age often develop greater confidence and resilience. Social interaction should be intentionally facilitated rather than assumed to develop passively, as it often does for sighted children. (8) Parents, teachers, and healthcare providers play an important role in this process and should be cautious not to impose unnecessary restrictions based on their own fears or assumptions about the child's vision. Instead, children should be encouraged to explore their abilities, discover their strengths, and learn their own limitations through experience.

Vision Loss and Reduced Quality of Life

While the factors described in this chapter can contribute to loneliness, withdrawal, and social isolation, these outcomes are not inevitable. Quality of life and emotional well-being after vision loss are complex and highly individual, shaped by multiple interacting factors. These include overall physical health, living situation, availability of supportive relationships, financial stability, access to resources, and opportunities for meaningful engagement.

Importantly, research shows that the degree of loneliness and depression experienced by individuals with vision loss is **not directly related to the severity of visual impairment.** (3) Rather, emotional well-being is more strongly influenced by how an individual accepts and adjusts to their vision loss, and by the supports available to help them adapt.

Vision rehabilitation services and peer support play an important role in this process. Rehabilitation programs help individuals understand and manage the functional and social challenges associated with vision loss, while fostering independence and confidence. Peer support and support groups offer a unique and powerful benefit: the opportunity to share experiences, normalize emotions, and learn practical coping strategies from others who truly understand the journey. These connections can significantly reduce feelings of loneliness and interrupt the progression toward social isolation.

Acceptance, Adjustment and Adaptation

The discussion of loneliness and social isolation brings us aback around to where the book started and the pillars of acceptance, adjustment, and adaptation.

Loneliness and social isolation following vision loss are not inevitable outcomes; rather, they often emerge when the emotional and practical work of acceptance, adjustment, and adaptation is interrupted or incomplete. These three processes form essential pillars that support continued connection to others and to the world. When one pillar is weakened, the risk of withdrawal, disengagement, and isolation increases.

Acceptance is the foundation. Without acknowledging the reality of vision loss, individuals may avoid social situations that expose visual limitations, withdraw from previously meaningful activities, or minimize their needs out of fear or embarrassment. Denial, while understandable, can quietly narrow a person's world. Avoided invitations, skipped outings, and reluctance to ask for assistance can gradually erode social networks. In contrast, acceptance allows individuals to acknowledge both loss and capability, opening the door to honest communication, self-compassion, and continued participation in relationships.

Adjustment builds upon acceptance by addressing the emotional and logistical changes that vision loss demands. As routines become more time-consuming and independence is redefined, frustration and fatigue can set in. Without adequate adjustment, individuals may feel burdensome or inadequate, reinforcing feelings of loneliness even when support is available. Successful adjustment, however, involves recalibrating expectations, recognizing personal limits without shame, and allowing others to assist when needed. This process preserves self-worth and helps maintain engagement in work, school, family life, and social roles.

Adaptation is where connection is actively restored and sustained. Through new skills, tools, and strategies—often supported by vision rehabilitation—individuals regain confidence in navigating their environment and participating in daily life. Adaptation reduces dependence-driven isolation by increasing functional independence and problem-solving ability. As confidence grows, so does willingness to re-enter social spaces, pursue hobbies, use technology to stay connected, and travel safely. Adaptation transforms vision loss from a barrier into a challenge that can be managed.

Together, acceptance, adjustment, and adaptation form a dynamic process that protects against loneliness and social isolation. They empower individuals not only to cope with vision loss, but to remain engaged, valued, and connected. By addressing both the emotional and practical dimensions of vision loss, these pillars support a life that remains socially meaningful—even as it is lived differently than before.

In the End...

If you are living with vision loss—or care about someone who is—it's important to understand that loneliness and social isolation are not simply the result of losing sight. They are shaped by many factors, including emotional well-being, confidence, relationships, and how supported a person feels by those around them. Vision loss affects far more than eyesight, and the challenges that follow are not only physical, but deeply psychological and social as well.

Recognizing these challenges is a powerful first step. Feelings of withdrawal, frustration, or isolation are not signs of weakness—they are common and understandable responses to major life change. Addressing social stigma, asking for support, and allowing time for acceptance, adjustment, and adaptation are essential parts of maintaining connection and emotional health. With understanding, appropriate support, and compassionate environments, it is possible to protect meaningful relationships and remain engaged in life. Vision loss may change how the world is experienced, but it does not have to mean facing that world alone.

References:

1. Rokach A., Berman D., Rose A. (2021). Loneliness of the blind and the visually impaired. *Frontiers in Psychology*, 12, Article 641711. https://doi.org/10.3389/fpsyg.2021.641711

2. Loneliness, social isolation and sight loss Research Findings Published by Thomas Pocklington Trust Dr Suzanne Hodge and Dr Fiona Eccles a

3. Klauke S, Sondocie C, Fine I. The impact of low vision on social function: The potential importance of lost visual social cues. J Optom. 2023 Jan-Mar;16(1):3-11. doi: 10.1016/j.optom.2022.03.003. Epub 2022 May 12. PMID: 35568628; PMCID: PMC9811370.

4. Royal National Institute of Blind People. (2017). *Employment status and sight loss*. https://www.rnib.org.uk/professionals/health-social-care-education-professionals/knowledge-and-research-hub/reports-and-insight/employment-status-and-sight-loss-2017/

5. Kong L., Gao Z., Xu N., Shao S., Ma H., He Q., Zhang D., Xu H., Qu H. (2021). The relation between self-stigma and loneliness in visually impaired college students: Self-acceptance as mediator. *Disability and Health Journal*, 14(2), Article 101054. https://doi.org/10.1016/j.dhjo.2020.101054

6. Bulk L. Y., Smith A., Nimmon L., Jarus T. (2020). A closer look at opportunities for blind adults: Impacts of stigmatization and ocularcentrism. *British Journal of Visual Impairment*, 38(3), 270–283. https://doi.org/10.1177/0264619620906942

7. Jackson SE, Hackett RA, Pardhan S, Smith L, Steptoe A. Association of Perceived Discrimination With Emotional Well-being in Older Adults With Visual Impairment. JAMA Ophthalmol. 2019 Jul 1;137(7):825-832. doi: 10.1001/jamaophthalmol.2019.1230. PMID: 31145413; PMCID: PMC6547384.

8. Sacks, S., Developing Social Skills in Children Who are Blind or Visually Impaired. Perkins School for the Blind, Resources.

The Americans with Disabilities Act and Low Vision

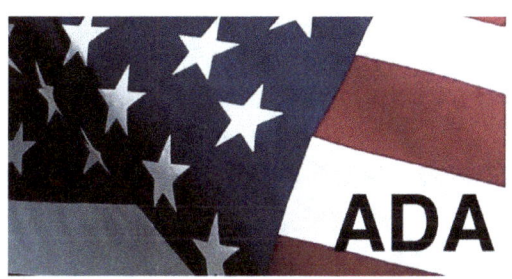

A Guide to Your Rights

The Americans with Disabilities Act (ADA) is a landmark federal civil rights law enacted in 1990 to prevent discrimination and guarantee equal opportunity for those with disabilities. It addresses equal access in employment, state and local government services, public accommodations, transportation, and telecommunications.

Prior to the ADA, individuals with disabilities lacked the comprehensive federal civil rights protections that existed for other groups. The law was set forth to help equalize social, economic, employment, and education disadvantages in the public domain.

Given the opportunity and appropriate accommodations, those with the disability of low vision can become full functioning, productive, and self-sufficient members of society.

Defining Disability and Vision Impairment

The ADA defines an individual with a disability using a three-pronged approach:

1. A person who has a physical or mental impairment that **substantially limits** one or more **major life activities** (like seeing, reading, or learning).

2. A person who has a **record** of such an impairment.

3. A person who is **regarded as** having such an impairment.

The ability to **see** is explicitly listed as a major life activity.

The Impact of the ADA Amendments Act (ADAAA)

The ADA was clarified and broadened by the ADA Amendments Act of 2008 (ADAAA). This is critical for people with low vision:

- **Mitigating Measures:** The determination of whether an impairment substantially limits a major life activity must generally be made **without regard to the ameliorative effects of mitigating measures.**

  This means the positive effects of **low-vision devices** (such as magnifiers, telescopes, and specialized computer software) must **not** be considered when determining if a person is disabled. If you need low-vision devices because of an underlying vision condition, that condition constitutes a disability.

- **Ordinary Eyeglasses/Contacts:** The one exception is for **ordinary eyeglasses or contact lenses** (lenses intended to fully correct visual acuity or eliminate refractive error). Their beneficial effects considered. Therefore, a person whose vision is fully corrected to the level of the general population using standard prescription lenses may not be considered disabled. However, if the underlying vision impairment still substantially limits the person's ability to see, even when using those lenses, or if the individual has an impairment that, in the absence of eyeglasses or contacts, substantially limits seeing, they meet the definition of disability.

It is important to note that while the ADA mandates accommodations, none of its provisions require entities to provide individuals with personal items such as eyeglasses, contact lenses, or other personal low-vision devices.

Employment (Title I)

Employment (Title I) Title I of the ADA prohibits discrimination in employment. This applies not just to hiring but also to job advancement, training, compensation, and "other terms, conditions, and privileges of employment."

- **Who Must Comply:** An employer must comply if they have **15 or more employees for each working day in each of 20 or more calendar weeks** in the current or preceding calendar year.

144

- **Qualified Individual:** The core protection is for a "**qualified individual on the basis of disability.**" A qualified person must be able to perform the **essential functions** of the job, with or without reasonable accommodations.

- **Reasonable Accommodation:** Employers must make "reasonable accommodation" for a disabled employee, providing there is no "undue hardship" for the employer. Hardship is determined based on cost, financial resources, the type of operation, and the overall impact on the facility.

Employer Tax Incentives

Federal law offers incentives to help employers offset the cost of accommodations.

- **Disabled Access Credit (Section 44):** Available to small businesses (those with $1 million or less in revenue or 30 or fewer full-time employees). It covers **50% of eligible access expenditures** between $250 and $10,250, with a maximum credit of $5,000 per year (50% of $10,000 = $5,000.).

- **Architectural/Transportation Barrier Removal Deduction (Section 190):** Available to all businesses for a maximum deduction of **$15,000** per year for expenses of removing qualified barriers.

  For more information, refer to the **U.S. Equal Employment Opportunity Commission (EEOC),** which enforces Title I. The document, Questions and Answers *About Visual Disabilities in the Workplace and the Americans with Disabilities Act, offers detailed guidance.*

Public Services (Title II)

Title II covers the programs, activities, and services of state and local government entities, regardless of their size or receipt of federal funds. This includes public education, transportation, health care, social services, courts, and voting.

- **The Mandate:** These entities must not discriminate against individuals with disabilities and must ensure their programs and services are accessible.

- **Accessibility and Communication:** For the visually impaired, this involves ensuring effective communication by providing auxiliary aids

145

and services at no additional cost. Examples include: qualified readers, accessible digital files, taped texts, Braille material, and large-print documents.

Education and Health Services Enforcement

- **Education:** The **U.S. Department of Education, Office for Civil Rights (OCR)**, enforces the education portion of the ADA, ensuring the rights and protection of students with disabilities. Modifications for qualified students—like time extensions, modified computers with text readers, or voice recognition software—must be reasonable and cannot fundamentally alter the program. However, educational institutions are not required to provide students with personal assistive devices.

U.S. Dept. of Education, OCR Contact	
Phone:	1-800-421-3481
TDD:	1-800-877-8339
Email:	ocr@ed.gov
Web Site:	https://www.ed.gov/ocr

- **Health and Social Programs:** The **U.S. Department of Health and Human Services (HHS), Office for Civil Rights**, enforces the health and social programs portion of Title II, ensuring non-exclusion from services offered by state and local government agencies.

Public Accommodations and Services Operated by Private Entities (Title III)

Title III addresses private-sector businesses and non-profit organizations that are open to the public, including places of lodging, restaurants, retail stores, movie theaters, private schools, and health care offices.

- **Exclusions:** Title III excludes private clubs and religious organizations.

- **Readily Achievable:** Covered entities must make **readily achievable** accommodations. This means "easily accomplishable and able to be carried out without much difficulty or expense," considering the entity's financial resources, the nature and cost of the action, and the size and type of business.

- **Communication:** Reasonable modifications to policies must be made to ensure access to goods and services. For the visually disabled, this is often about communication, such as having an employee read a menu or price information. For more complex documents (contracts, forms), the visually disabled have the right to request access via alternate formats, such as computer disc, audio, or email.

- **Signage:** The ADA Standards for Accessible Design, Chapter 7, details requirements for permanent signage (restrooms, room identifiers, exits). This includes specifications for Braille, tactile (raised lettering), visual contrast, and sign location.

The **U.S. Department of Justice (DOJ), Civil Rights Division**, enforces both Title II and Title III of the ADA.

147

U.S. Department of Justice Contact	
Disability Rights Section	Civil Rights Division, U.S. Department of Justice,' P.O. Box 66738, Washington D.C., 20035-6738
Toll-Free:	1-800-514-0301
TTY:	1-800-514-0383

Summary

The ADA has evolved through court rulings and modifications, notably the ADAAA, which ensured broad coverage for those with impairments, including low vision. Its ultimate goal is to eliminate prejudice, prevent exclusion and segregation, and act as an equalizer. Those with disabilities, including low vision, should be able to move about freely and enjoy all the privileges and advantages available to others.

Understanding Macular Degeneration

The 7 Truths about Age -Related Macular Degeneration

While your risk for age-related macular degeneration (AMD) increases as you get older, it is neither inevitable nor necessarily blinding. Although there is no cure, there are effective strategies for prevention and treatment. A diagnosis of AMD is not the end of your independence or quality of life—there is hope, help, and a path forward.

Truth #1 The risk for developing macular degeneration increases with age.

Population studies have consistently demonstrated a correlation between visual acuity and age, revealing a higher prevalence of vision impairment and legal blindness as individuals grow older. This trend is most pronounced among those aged 65 and above, with a notable escalation in incidence beyond the age of 75.

According to data from the Centers for Disease Control and Prevention (CDC), an estimated 19.8 million Americans aged 40 and above are affected by some form of age-related macular degeneration. (1) A figure that rises to 67 million across the European Union. AMD stands as the primary cause of permanent vision impairments among individuals over 65, with a particularly elevated occurrence among those of European descent. (2)

The World Health Organization (WHO) approximates that the United States witnesses 200,000 new cases of AMD annually, while Europe experiences 400,000 new cases per year. Projections from the WHO indicate a global population of 196 million individuals with AMD in 2020, with an anticipated increase in cases by 2040, bringing the total to 288 million cases worldwide. (3)

With our population aging, there is a proportional rise in the percentage of older age cohorts. Consequently, research indicates a forthcoming surge in the number of individuals grappling with vision impairments. Addressing these challenges falls within the purview of low vision rehabilitation, a specialized field within vision care.

Truth #2 Macular degeneration is not inevitable as we age.

The progression of vision loss associated with aging, such as macular degeneration, is not an inevitable fate. While maintaining good vision as we age is indeed achievable, numerous factors come into play that can influence the health of our eyes and overall well-being. Macular degeneration, in particular, is a complex condition influenced by various factors including general health, genetics, and environmental elements.

Research consistently demonstrates a strong link between overall health and eye health. Nutrition, in particular, is a powerful modifiable factor. Diets rich in protective nutrients—such as antioxidants, carotenoids, and omega-3 fatty acids—have been shown to support retinal function and may slow the progression of macular degeneration. Certain nutritional supplements have also been clinically proven to help stabilize or even modestly reverse early stages of the disease.

In addition, the interaction between genetics and environmental factors is now better understood. Our genes, encoded within DNA, do not act in isolation. Environmental exposures—such as UV radiation, smoking, medication use, or dietary toxins—can influence the expression of these genes. This interaction can either protect against or contribute to the onset of degenerative eye diseases like macular degeneration, glaucoma, or cataracts.

Regular exercise is also fundamental to promoting overall health, as it enhances blood vessel flexibility and circulation. This ensures adequate oxygenation and nutrient delivery to the delicate blood vessels of the eye, supporting their optimal function.

Moreover, prioritizing routine eye examinations is important. Early detection of eye diseases, coupled with expert guidance from a responsive eye care professional, can significantly impact the prognosis of these conditions.

Ultimately, the choices we make regarding diet and lifestyle significantly influence how we age. By adopting a proactive approach to eye health through proper nutrition, exercise, and regular check-ups, we empower ourselves to maintain optimal vision and overall well-being as we navigate the aging process.

Truth #3 It is not inevitable that those with macular degeneration will go blind.

Macular degeneration is a leading cause of vision impairment, but it does not inevitably result in complete blindness. The degree of vision loss can vary widely from person to person, and many individuals retain useful peripheral vision even in the advanced stages of the disease. Importantly, how blindness is defined plays an important role in how we understand the impact of macular degeneration.

Is macular degeneration considered legal blindness?

The American Medical Association developed a clinical definition of blindness that has since been adopted by government agencies such as the Social Security Administration and state disability programs. Many individuals with age-related macular degeneration qualify for state or federal assistance due to their classification as "legally blind."

According to these guidelines, *legal blindness* is defined as having a visual acuity of 20/200 (6/60) or worse in the better eye, even when using the best possible corrective lenses. Another criterion is having a visual field of 20 degrees or less. However, legal blindness does not equate to total blindness or complete loss of sight—it simply indicates a level of vision that significantly impairs daily functioning.

> *The Social Security Administration no longer uses the designation
> 'legally blind.' They now use the term 'statutory blindness.'

Our ability to perceive visual acuity relies on the densely packed sensory neurons in the central vision area. This region, characterized by a high concentration of neurons, is particularly susceptible to fluctuations in oxygen and nutrient levels. Consequently, it is the central area of acute vision that is most profoundly affected by various health and environmental factors.

Consider the nature of age-related macular degeneration: It entails the progressive degeneration of the central macular area of vision leading to diminished visual acuity. The peripheral vision typically remains intact. While reading, recognizing faces, and driving may become difficult or impossible, individuals with AMD rarely lose all vision.

153

The Stages of Macular Degeneration.

There are stages to 'dry' macular degeneration. It is only the final advanced stages that results in 'legal blindness.' 90% of those diagnosed with macular degeneration have the dry form. 10% go on to the vision devastating 'wet' form of macular degeneration.

Early 'Dry macular degeneration:

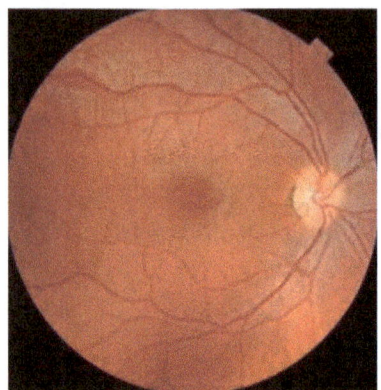 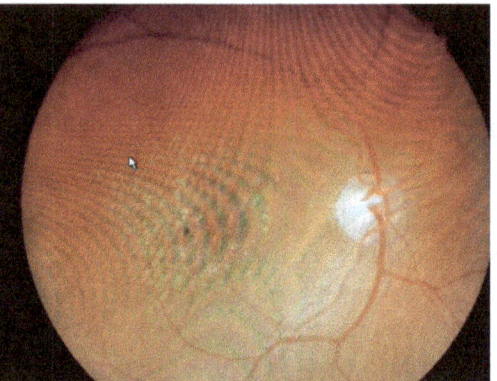

Normal retina: Macula with drusen
central macula and optic nerve

- Developed slowly,
- characterized by white small deposits called drusen,
- causes some visual acuity loss: 20/20 to 20/40 (6/6 to6/12).

Intermediate 'dry' macular degeneration:

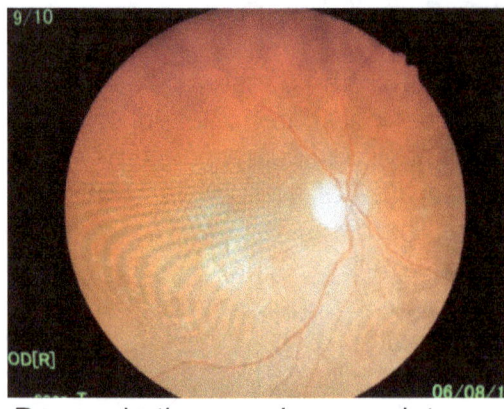

- Slow, progression continues,
- accumulation of more and larger drusen,
- more visual acuity loss; 20/40 to 20/100 (6/12 to 6/30).

Drusen in the macular area, intermediate Dry AMD

Advanced 'dry' macular degeneration:

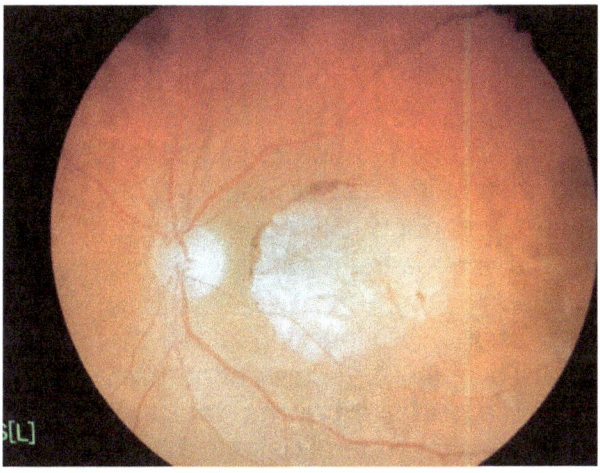

Atrophic 'dry' macular degeneration;

• End stage of 'dry' macular degeneration,
• death of the retinal cells of the macula, resulting in **geographic atrophy**,
• visual acuity, less than 20/200 (6/60), 'legally blind.'

Geographic atrophy, cells of the macula have died, resulting in central vision loss.

Wet Macular Degeneration

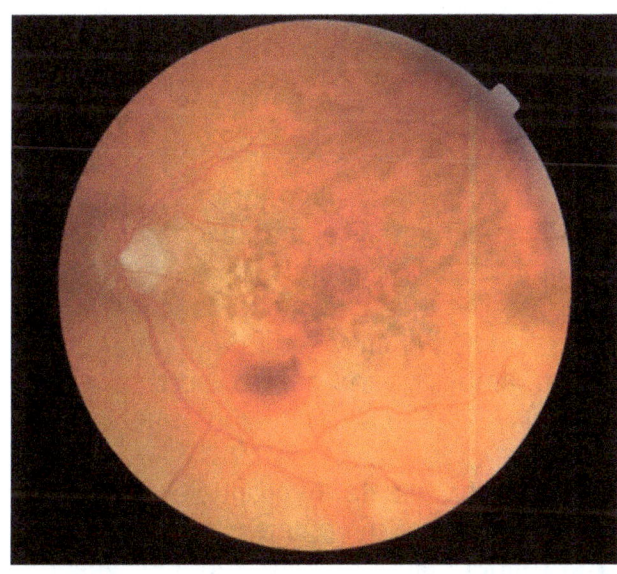

'Wet' macular degeneration;

•   A sudden, rapid loss of central vision,
•   inflammatory process, characterized by leakage and bleeding of blood vessels beneath the macula, resulting in scarring.
•   Most severe devastating loss of vision, visual acuity, less than 20/200 (6/60).

'Wet' macular degeneration characterized by leakage and bleeding.

155

Can You still see with Macular Degeneration?

Macular degeneration is often associated with the fear of total vision loss in older adults. However, in most cases, significant residual vision remains.

Although the macula—the central part of the retina responsible for sharp, detailed vision—is compromised, the rest of the retina usually continues to function. Peripheral vision remains intact, although it is not as sharp due to a lower concentration of photoreceptor cells outside the macula.

The key to maximizing remaining vision lies in learning to use the healthier areas surrounding the damaged macula. Techniques such as **eccentric fixation**, also known as **eccentric viewing** or using a **preferred retinal locus (PRL)**, can help individuals adapt by relying on these alternate retinal regions for visual tasks.

Truth# 4 There is no cure for macular degeneration.

Just as there is no cure for the natural changes that accompany aging, there remains no definitive cure for age-related macular degeneration (AMD). While many cells in the body have the remarkable ability to regenerate throughout life, the same cannot be said for the delicate and highly specialized cells of the retina.

The retinal pigment epithelium (RPE) plays an important role in supporting both the photoreceptors (the light-sensing cells) and the underlying blood vessel layer. Unfortunately, RPE cells have a limited ability to replicate. As we age, their number and function gradually decline. Ideally, these cells should last a lifetime, but various harmful factors—such as oxidative stress, inadequate nutrition, excessive ultraviolet (UV) light exposure, smoking, and genetic predisposition—can accelerate their damage or death.

When RPE cells begin to deteriorate, waste byproducts from retinal metabolism accumulate in the form of **drusen.** Over time, this buildup, along with the progressive loss of both RPE and retinal cells, leads to impaired vision. At present, there is no way to regenerate these cells once they are lost.

Still, while a cure remains out of reach, there are important advances in managing the disease. Treatments such as **anti-VEGF** (anti-**V**ascular **E**ndothelial **G**rowth **F**actor) injections for wet AMD, lifestyle modifications and nutritional support, can help preserve remaining vision and slow progression. Additionally, emerging research in areas like stem cell therapy, retinal implants, and gene therapy offers hope for the future.

Truth #5. There are treatments available.

A diagnosis of macular degeneration can feel overwhelming, but it's important to understand that various treatments and strategies now exist to help manage the condition—whether it's the more common slowly, progressive dry form or the more severe wet form. While there is still no cure, both lifestyle changes and medical interventions can help preserve vision and reduce progression.

Let's first explore the more prevalent form:

Dry age-related macular degeneration (AMD).

Managing Dry AMD: Slowing Progression Through Lifestyle and Nutrition

There is currently no medical cure for dry AMD, largely due to its complex origins involving genetics, aging, systemic health, and environmental stressors. However, that doesn't mean you're powerless. The goal of treatment here is to **slow progression**, reduce the risk of complications such as geographic atrophy, and support overall retinal health.

The body faces many stressors as we age—pollutants, UV radiation, heavy metals, and oxidative byproducts of metabolism—all of which contribute to **oxidative stress**, a key factor in AMD. This is where dietary changes and targeted supplementation play a powerful role.

A nutrient-rich diet—especially one high in fruits and vegetables—offers a natural defense through antioxidants. Numerous studies have shown that people who consume diets rich in antioxidants, vitamins, and carotenoids have a **lower risk** of developing AMD or seeing it worsen.

To enhance this protective effect, supplementation is often recommended. **The Age-Related Eye Disease Study (AREDS)** found that a specific blend of vitamins and antioxidants slowed the progression of intermediate to advanced AMD by about 25%. Although more details on the AREDS formulation are

157

covered in my book on ocular health, it's worth noting here that vitamins C and E, along with lutein, zeaxanthin, and zinc, are key players in defending retinal cells from damage.

In addition to general supplements, patients with geographic atrophy—an advanced form of dry AMD—may now benefit from in-office treatments.

Geographic Atrophy: New Medical Options for Dry AMD

In 2023, the FDA approved two treatments for **geographic atrophy (GA)**: intravitreal injections designed to slow progression of this advanced stage of dry AMD. (4) While these injections do not reverse damage already done, they can preserve existing vision for longer by slowing the disease's course. Treatment is tailored to the individual and should be discussed with a retina specialist.

When Dry AMD Becomes Wet: Anti-VEGF and Other In-Office Treatments

About 10% of patients with dry AMD progress to the wet form—also known as **neovascular AMD**. Though less common, this form accounts for 85% of AMD-related legal blindness due to the aggressive nature of abnormal blood vessel growth beneath the macula.

These fragile, leaky vessels develop in response to low oxygen levels in the retina and can lead to sudden vision loss. Prompt detection and treatment are critical.

The main treatment for wet AMD is anti-VEGF therapy, which blocks the vascular endothelial growth factor responsible for triggering new, abnormal blood vessels.

There are currently three main treatment approaches:

1. **Anti-VEGF Injections** (anti-**V**ascular **E**ndothelial **G**rowth **F**actor)
   A medication is injected directly into the eye every 4 to 8 weeks. This medication halts the growth of abnormal vessels and often stabilizes or even improves vision. Common drugs include Avastin, Lucentis, Eylea, and Beovu.
2. **Photodynamic Therapy (PDT)**
   Less commonly used today, this involves an injection of Visudyne® into the arm. The drug accumulates in abnormal vessels, which are then targeted with a cold laser to seal them off. PDT may still be helpful in

cases where anti-VEGF therapy isn't an option or needs to be supplemented.

3. **Combination Therapy**
In some cases, anti-VEGF and PDT are combined to optimize outcomes.

These procedures are performed in a retina specialist's office on an outpatient basis and typically require regular follow-up.

Final Thoughts

Macular degeneration is a progressive disease, but not an untreatable one. With early detection, a healthy lifestyle, and access to modern therapies, it is increasingly possible to preserve functional vision and maintain quality of life. The road may require ongoing care and adjustments, but patients have more tools than ever before.

Truth #6 AMD is preventable.

Age-related macular degeneration develops over a lifetime—often due to cumulative wear and tear, and sometimes, from habits that place unnecessary stress on the body. The encouraging truth is this: for many individuals already diagnosed with AMD, further progression of the disease is not inevitable. With proper care, lifestyle modifications, and awareness, it can be slowed—or in some cases, potentially halted.

1. Healthy Body, Healthy Eyes

Macular degeneration often occurs in individuals who have other underlying health concerns. Conditions such as **hypertension**, **nutritional deficiencies** (whether from poor diet or poor digestion), **cardiovascular disease**, and **diabetes** have all been associated with a higher risk of AMD. By addressing these systemic health issues, you reduce the risk of both developing AMD and worsening it.

Keep in mind: **some high blood pressure medications** can deplete the body of water-soluble vitamins and minerals. If you take such medications, speak with your healthcare provider about whether nutritional supplementation is appropriate.

2. Eat Well and Supplement When Needed

Prioritize a diet rich in **fruits and vegetables**, which provide antioxidants and essential nutrients for retinal health. Include **fatty fish**, such as salmon, sardines, or mackerel, for their omega-3 content. If you don't eat fish, consider supplementing with **DHA and EPA** (marine-sourced omega-3s) or **flaxseed oil** (a plant-based source).

Avoid **processed vegetable oils**, such as generic vegetable oil and corn oil, which are often refined and pro-inflammatory. Instead, use **cold-pressed, unrefined oils** like olive oil or avocado oil.

Also, reduce intake of **processed foods**, **refined sugars**, and **white flour**, which are low in nutrients and can contribute to inflammation and metabolic dysfunction.

A **heart-healthy diet** supports not just cardiovascular wellness—it promotes eye health as well.

3. Stop Smoking

Smoking introduces toxic chemicals into the bloodstream that damage blood vessels and retinal tissue. Research has shown that **smoking can double the risk of developing AMD**. If you smoke, quitting is one of the most impactful steps you can take to protect your vision. (5)

4. Protect Your Eyes from UV and Blue Light

Chronic exposure to **ultraviolet (UV)** and **high-energy visible blue light** is believed to contribute to the development of AMD. UV radiation can trigger **photochemical damage** to eye tissues, and eyes already affected by disease may be even more vulnerable.

UVA and UVB rays can penetrate cloud cover and reach the eyes even on overcast days. Wearing **UV-protective sunglasses** and wide-brimmed hats whenever you're outdoors is a simple, effective way to reduce your lifetime exposure.

5. Get Regular Exercise

The benefits of **physical activity** extend far beyond weight control. Regular aerobic exercise reduces the risk of **cardiovascular disease** and supports **cognitive function**—both of which are closely tied to ocular health.

Exercise increases blood flow to the eyes, enhancing delivery of **oxygen and nutrients** to the retina and surrounding structures.

The American Heart Association recommends: (6)

- **At least 150 minutes per week** of moderate-intensity aerobic activity (e.g., brisk walking),
  or
- **75 minutes per week** of vigorous aerobic activity (e.g., running), *preferably spread throughout the week.*
- In addition, include **muscle-strengthening activities** (such as weight training or resistance work) on **at least two days per week**.

6. Know Your Risk Factors

Understanding your personal risk profile can empower you to make informed choices. The most significant risk factors for AMD include:

- Advancing age
- Family history of AMD
- Smoking
- Hypertension

Other contributing risk factors include:

- Diets high in **refined vegetable oils**
- Excessive **fat intake**, especially processed mono- and polyunsaturated fatty acids
- Diets rich in **white flour-based foods**
- Having **light-colored irises** (e.g., blue eyes)

While not all risk factors can be controlled, many can. A focus on **a healthful diet**, **consistent lifestyle choices**, and **medical awareness** can go a long way toward preserving your sight.

161

Truth #7 Life does not end with the diagnosis of macular degeneration.

To many, the term *low vision* remains unclear, while *legally blind* is more widely recognized. In reality, low vision encompasses a broad range of visual impairment that cannot be fully corrected with glasses, contact lenses, medication, or surgery. It is more meaningful to define it based on **functional vision**—how effectively a person uses their remaining sight to perform daily activities.

Vision rehabilitation aims to help individuals maximize their remaining vision and reclaim independence. This collaborative process with eye care professionals and rehabilitation specialists empowers people to improve quality of life—not by restoring lost vision, but by strengthening their ability to function with what they still have.

Today, more resources are available than ever before. It is, in many ways, the best time in history to live with low vision.

The adaptation process typically begins with identifying specific challenges and then building a personalized plan around four key areas:

1. Medical Management

The role of optometrists, ophthalmologists, and primary care providers is crucial. They diagnose and monitor the disease, identify risk factors, and manage associated health concerns. Regular eye exams are essential, along with maintaining a treatment regimen tailored to your needs.

Lifestyle changes are often advised—especially diet, exercise, and smoking cessation. A healthy body supports a healthy brain and healthy eyes.

2. Counseling and Support

Vision loss affects more than eyesight. Therapists and counselors can address psychological and emotional concerns, provide guidance, and connect individuals with resources such as state services, rehabilitation programs, and financial support.

These professionals help individuals and families cope with the emotional impact of vision loss—and remind them that they are not alone in the journey.

3. Non-Optical Aids for Daily Living

Simple daily activities—cooking, grooming, shopping, cleaning, managing medications—can become frustrating. These tasks, known as *activities of daily living* (ADLs), can be made easier with basic adjustments:

- Improved lighting
- High-contrast color cues
- Tactile identifiers
- Talking devices
- Organizational strategies

Occupational therapists are instrumental in this process. They provide home and workplace evaluations and offer hands-on training in both non-optical and optical solutions.

4. Optical Devices and Low Vision Tools

Rehabilitation often begins with an optimal prescription for glasses. But for tasks that require detail—such as reading, writing, or hobbies—magnification becomes essential. This may include:

- Handheld or stand magnifiers
- Telescopes
- Video magnifiers
- Wearable visual aids

Low vision specialists help assess your needs and guide you toward the most appropriate devices. Occupational therapists then train you in their effective use.

5. Assistive Technology and Smart Tools

Technology has opened a new frontier for those with vision loss. Today's smartphones and tablets offer built-in accessibility features such as:

- Screen magnification
- Text-to-speech

- High contrast modes
- Voice commands

Apps can assist with navigation, identify objects, read text aloud, or magnify printed material.

Voice-controlled virtual assistants—like Alexa, Siri, or Google Assistant—allow users to check the weather, send messages, or control smart home devices entirely by voice. When paired with smart technology, they can manage lighting, security, reminders, and more—without relying on vision.

A diagnosis of macular degeneration may feel like an ending—but it can also be a beginning. With guidance, training, and support, individuals can redefine what is possible. **The path forward lies not in recovering what was lost, but in learning how to live fully with what remains.**

Acceptance. Adjustment. Adaptation. These are the pillars of resilience—and the foundation for a meaningful life after vision loss.

In the End...

While some aspects of macular degeneration lie beyond our control—such as genetics or age—many others can be influenced through lifestyle, medical care, and informed choices. Success in living well with macular degeneration begins with knowledge, but it doesn't end there. A willingness to learn, to accept what cannot be changed, and to actively adjust and adapt to new realities is what ultimately shapes your experience.

With the right support, tools, and mindset, it is entirely possible to maintain independence, preserve meaningful vision, and live a full and rewarding life.

In the following chapters, we'll explore more tools, technologies, and daily strategies to help you adapt and thrive with changing vision.

"The pessimist complains about the wind. The optimist expects it to change. The leader adjusts the sails." John C. Maxwell

References

1. Rein DB, Wittenborn JS, Burke-Conte Z, Gulia R, Robalik T, Ehrlich JR, Lundeen EA, Flaxman AD. Prevalence of Age-Related Macular Degeneration in the US in 2019. JAMA Ophthalmol. 2022 Dec 1;140(12):1202-1208. doi:

2. National Eye Institute. 2010 U.S. age-specific prevalence rates for AMD by age and race/ethnicity.

3. World Health Organization. World Report on Vision, Executive Summary.

4. 2025 American Macular Degeneration Foundation **FDA Approves First Geographic Atrophy Treatment, SYFOVRE**

5. Vingerling JR, Hofman A, Grobbee DE, de Jong PT. Age-related macular degeneration and smoking. The Rotterdam Study. Arch Ophthalmol. 1996 Oct;114(10):1193-6. doi: 10.1001/archopht.

6. American Heart Association. American Heart Association Recommendations for Physical Activity in Adults and Kids. Last Reviewed: Jan 19, 2024

Seeing Through Macular Degeneration

Macular degeneration primarily affects central vision while typically sparing peripheral vision. As a result, individuals with this condition often retain some degree of functional sight, particularly for tasks that do not rely heavily on sharp, central focus.

To navigate the challenges of central vision loss, many people use a combination of visual aids, assistive technologies, and adaptive techniques. These may include magnifying lenses, electronic magnifiers, screen-reading software, and a method called eccentric viewing—training the eyes to use healthier areas of the retina to compensate for central vision loss. These tools and strategies can make everyday tasks more manageable and help maintain a level of independence.

When the Center Fades: Visual Perception with Macular Degeneration

The visual experience of someone with macular degeneration depends on whether they have the dry or wet form of the disease, as well as the stage of its progression. No two individuals will experience the condition in exactly the same way. Some changes occur gradually, while others can develop suddenly—particularly in the case of wet macular degeneration.

Here are some common ways that people with macular degeneration may perceive their surroundings:

Blurred Vision:

In the early stages, mild blurriness is often one of the first signs. This blurring usually affects the central vision and may be mistaken for the need for a stronger eyeglass prescription. However, when examined by an eye care professional, a new prescription does not improve the clarity. This is often the first clue that something more serious is occurring in the retina.

Metamorphopsia:

This visual distortion is also an early sign of macular degeneration. Metamorphopsia refers to the **perception of warped or misshapen** objects. Straight lines may appear wavy or bent, and printed text may look jumbled or uneven. These distortions can make reading and recognizing faces particularly difficult, even when visual acuity seems relatively unchanged.

Twenty miles offshore in the cool California current, the park includes five of the eight remarkable Channel Islands: San Miguel, Santa Rosa, Santa Cruz (*the largest*), Anacapa, and Santa Barbara. Isolated for thousands of years, 145 of the 2,000 species of plants and animals that live on these islands—a UNESCO biosphere reserve—exist nowhere else on Earth. A few species, such as the island scrub jay and the Santa Cruz Island silver lotus, are found only on Santa Cruz.

A human skeleton found on Santa Rosa Island was dated to more than 13,000 years ago—the oldest human remains found in North America. Woolly mammoth fos-

Twenty miles offshore in the cool California current, the park includes five of the eight remarkable Channel Islands: San Miguel, Santa Rosa, Santa Cruz (the largest), Anacapa, and Santa Barbara. Isolated for thousands of years, 145 of the 2,000 species of plants and animals, on these islands—a UNESCO biosphere reserve, else on Earth. A few species, such as the island silver lotus, are found *only* on Santa Cruz.

A human skeleton found on Santa Rosa Island was dated to more than 13,000 years ago—the oldest human remains found in North America. Woolly mammoth fos-

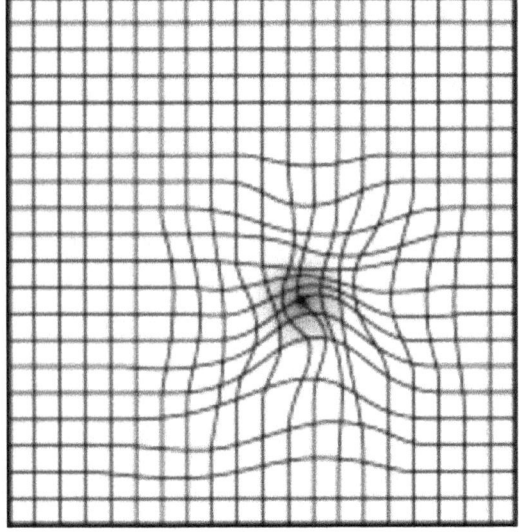

Metamorphopsia, the distortion seen with macular degeneration. The Amsler grid used to detect distortion and monitor for changes.

As macular degeneration advances, the number and size of drusen increase, along with pigment changes in the retina. These changes lead to more significant central vision loss. The decline may occur gradually, but it often becomes increasingly noticeable and disruptive, especially for tasks that depend on sharp central vision.

Central Blind Spot

In later stages, individuals may experience a pronounced central blind spot. This loss of central vision interferes with activities like reading, recognizing faces, and driving—tasks that demand high-resolution visual detail.

Interestingly, people with macular degeneration do not say that they see a "hole" in their vision, black, grey, or otherwise. The brain has this great capability to 'fill in' the space. However, it can't see what it can't see, meaning it will fill in with the background colors of the surrounding area.

Despite the central vision loss, peripheral vision typically remains functional. This preserved peripheral vision enables individuals to navigate their environment and engage in activities that don't require fine detail.

The loss of central vision doesn't mean the end of reading. With the right tools and strategies, many individuals can continue to enjoy books, articles, and even digital content—just in new ways.

Reading with Macular Degeneration: Tools and Techniques

Reading can become difficult for individuals with macular degeneration, especially in the more advanced stages when central vision is significantly affected. However, there are many strategies and assistive technologies that can help people continue to access written materials:

1. **Magnifying Reading Glasses**
   Specialized reading glasses with built-in magnification may be prescribed to enhance near vision. However, there is a practical limit to how much magnification can be used comfortably without causing eye strain or reducing the field of view.

2. **Optical Magnification Devices**
   Familiar tools like handheld or stand magnifiers are widely available and relatively affordable. These optical devices enlarge print and images and can be useful for short reading tasks. Modified telescopes can also be adapted for near-vision reading in some cases.

169

3. **Electronic Magnifiers**
   Digital magnifiers—also known as video magnifiers or closed-circuit television (CCTV) systems—use a camera to display text on a screen with adjustable magnification and contrast. These devices are especially helpful for extended reading sessions or materials with small print.

4. **Large Print Materials**
   Books, magazines, and newspapers in large print are easier to read for those with mild vision loss. When combined with a magnifier, large print materials can greatly improve readability and comfort.

5. **Audiobooks and Text-to-Speech Technology**
   Listening to books through audiobooks or using software that converts text into speech can reduce eye fatigue and increase reading speed. These alternatives are ideal for individuals who struggle with visual reading or who experience discomfort with magnification devices.

6. **Accessibility Features on Mobile Devices**
   Enlarging the font on smartphones or tablets may not be enough. Fortunately, most devices come with built-in accessibility settings, such as text-to-speech options. There are also mobile apps that read on-screen text aloud and even offer speech-to-text features—allowing users to dictate messages and emails. These tools can significantly improve digital communication, even if the occasional speech-to-text error adds a bit of humor.

7. **Braille**
   For individuals with profound or progressive vision loss, learning Braille offers a tactile method of reading. While not necessary for everyone, it can be a valuable option for those who are no longer able to read visually.

With the right tools, strategies, and support, many people with macular degeneration can continue to enjoy reading and maintain their connection to the written word.

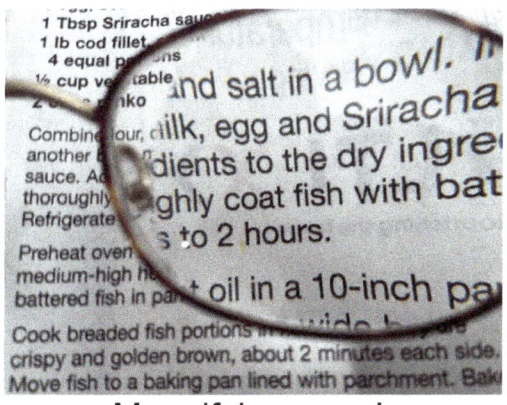

Magnifying eyeglasses

Hand-held magnifiers

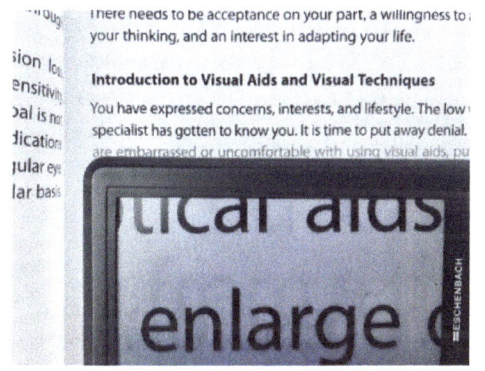

Video magnifiers

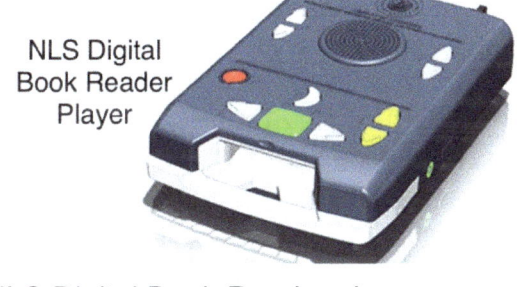

NLS Digital Book Reader Player

NLS Digital Book Reader player

Magnification Beyond Reading:

Tools for Seeing the World with Macular Degeneration for Distance Vision Tools: Telescopes and Smart Glasses for Low Vision

While magnification is often associated with reading aids, it can also support many other aspects of daily life for individuals with macular degeneration. Specialized optical and digital devices—such as **telescopes and smart glasses**—can significantly enhance distance vision, orientation, and overall engagement with the environment.

171

Telescopes: Bringing the Distance Closer

Distance Viewing:
Telescopic devices can enlarge distant objects, making it easier to recognize faces, read street signs, or watch television—tasks that often become difficult with central vision loss.

Intermittent Use for Spotting:
Some telescopes are designed for brief, targeted use. A user may raise the telescope to identify details—like writing on a whiteboard or a presentation screen—and then move it aside. This makes them useful for quick visual tasks without needing to wear them continuously.

Outdoor Activities and Events:
Telescopes can enhance recreational experiences such as bird watching, stargazing, or enjoying sporting events. When accessibility features like large screens or audio descriptions aren't available, telescopes can provide a direct view of the action.

Orientation and Navigation:
For individuals navigating unfamiliar areas, telescopes can help identify landmarks or read building signs from a distance. This can make sightseeing, travel, or simply walking through a city more manageable.

Smart Glasses: Digital Vision Enhancement

Smart glasses are an advanced alternative to traditional telescopes, offering real-time magnification through built-in cameras and digital displays. These wearable devices do more than just enlarge images—they integrate assistive technology in a compact, hands-free format.

Visual and Text Magnification:
Smart glasses can magnify the user's surroundings, often with adjustable zoom. Some models include optical character recognition and text-to-speech technology (OCR/TTS), which converts printed word into an on-screen display (OCR) or reads printed text aloud (TTS)—helpful for reading signs, menus, or product labels.

Connectivity and Features:
Many smart glasses connect to smartphones or tablets via Bluetooth or Wi-Fi, giving users access to voice assistants, apps, and touch-free control options.

172

GPS capabilities in some models provide spoken navigation cues, aiding independent travel.

Training and Accessibility:
Although smart glasses offer greater functionality than standard telescopes, they may require more technical skill to operate. Some manufacturers provide in-person or online training to help users become comfortable with the technology. It's also important to consider the higher cost of these devices when choosing between options.

Personalized Tools for Better Vision

Both telescopes and smart glasses belong to a growing range of assistive technologies designed to help those with visual impairments remain independent and engaged in everyday life. The right solution depends on the user's individual needs, lifestyle, and comfort with technology. A low vision specialist can help evaluate which tools will offer the greatest benefit.

While magnification is often associated with reading, it can also play an important role in helping individuals with macular degeneration manage other everyday activities more independently.

Telescopes

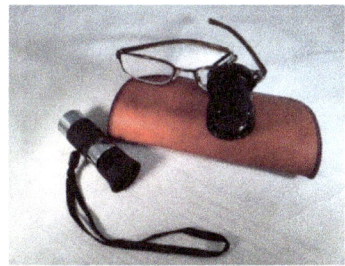 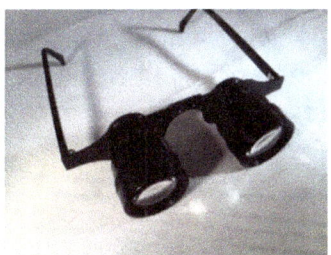 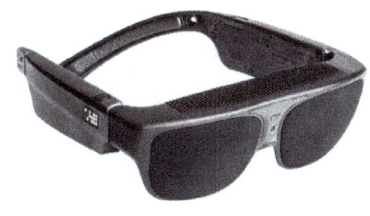

Hand-held and mounted   Low vision binoculars   eSight smart glasses

Shifting Focus: Eccentric Viewing for Macular Degeneration

Eccentric viewing is a technique used by individuals with macular degeneration or other forms of central vision loss to make better use of their remaining peripheral vision. It is especially helpful for tasks that typically depend on central vision, such as reading, recognizing faces, or watching television.

This adaptive strategy involves consciously directing the gaze away from the central blind spot to a healthier part of the retina—often in the peripheral field. By learning to shift their focus to these areas, individuals can capture visual information more effectively, despite damage to the macula.

For reading, this may involve looking slightly above, below, or to the side of the text rather than directly at it. Through practice, individuals can locate a "preferred retinal locus" (PRL)—the spot on the peripheral retina that provides the clearest image—and train themselves to use it consistently. This may also require repositioning the reading material or using magnifiers to enlarge the text within the PRL's range.

Eccentric viewing is not limited to reading. It can also be applied to everyday visual tasks like recognizing faces, preparing food, navigating the environment, or watching television. When combined with assistive devices—such as optical magnifiers, electronic magnifiers, or wearable technologies—eccentric viewing strategies can significantly improve functional vision.

Training in eccentric viewing is typically provided through **low vision rehabilitation programs**. Vision specialists work closely with individuals to tailor techniques based on their unique pattern of vision loss, needs, and goals. As with all aspects of low vision therapy, the success of eccentric viewing depends on personalized training and regular practice.

Eccentric viewing is just one part of a comprehensive approach to managing vision loss. With the right tools, strategies, and professional support, individuals with central vision impairment can improve their ability to perform everyday tasks and maintain their independence.

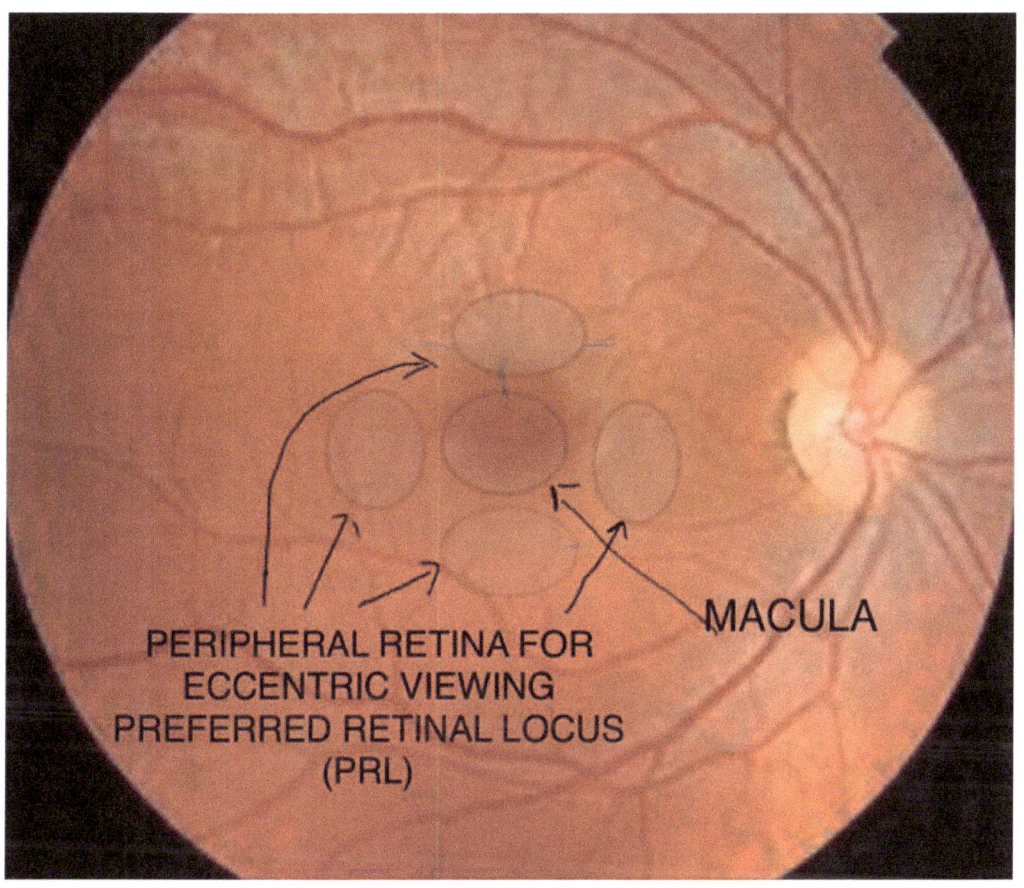

Retina of a right eye, indicating the central macular area and the peripheral areas of the retina used for eccentric viewing.

In the End...

Macular degeneration can significantly affect daily life, but techniques like eccentric viewing—along with the use of visual aids and guidance from low vision specialists—can help individuals maximize their remaining vision. Regular eye examinations are essential for tracking changes in vision and receiving timely recommendations. If you or someone you know is experiencing vision changes, consult an eye care professional for a comprehensive evaluation.

How To Monitor for Progression of Macular Degeneration

The Amsler grid has long been the standard self-monitoring tool for detecting changes in vision due to eye disease. While still useful, newer technologies—such as smartphone apps and home monitoring devices—can offer more precise and timely detection of changes in vision.

Self-monitoring is especially important for:

1. Individuals at risk for developing sight-threatening eye conditions,
2. early detection of vision changes caused by eye disease, and
3. tracking the progression of conditions such as macular degeneration and diabetic eye disease.

Dry age-related macular degeneration (AMD) typically progresses slowly, often with subtle changes in vision. Because these changes can go unnoticed, especially in the early stages, self-monitoring plays a key role in catching signs of deterioration that might otherwise be missed.

Wet AMD, by contrast, is a more aggressive and potentially vision-threatening form of the disease. About 10% to 15% of individuals with dry AMD will progress to this faster-developing stage. If your eye care provider has identified you as having macular degeneration—or as being at risk for developing wet AMD—there are now home-based technologies designed specifically to detect both gradual changes in dry AMD and the sudden onset of wet AMD. The earlier treatment begins, the greater the chance of preventing catastrophic vision loss.

The Amsler Grid: A Simple Tool for Detecting Vision Changes

Anyone diagnosed with age-related macular degeneration should be familiar with the Amsler Grid. This simple, low-cost tool allows individuals to monitor their central vision at home and detect early signs of disease progression, particularly within the central 20 degrees of the visual field.

Typically provided by an eye care professional, the Amsler Grid is a printed square pattern—usually on a card or sheet of paper—with a central dot. While basic, this grid remains a valuable method for observing subtle changes in the macula that may indicate worsening AMD.

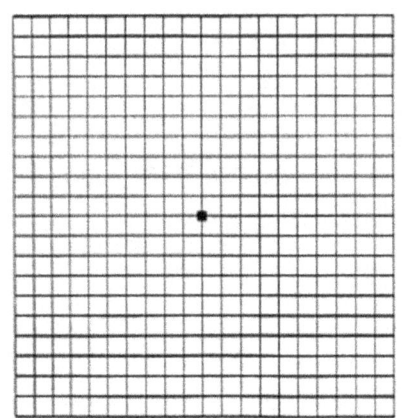 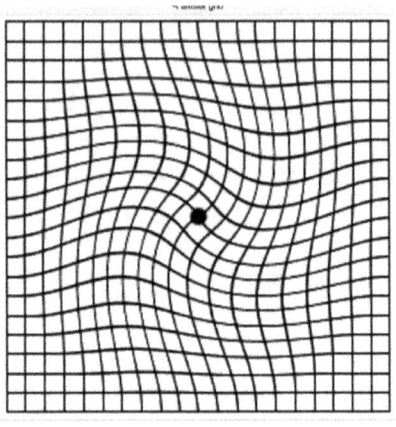

Normal appearance of Amsler grid   Distortion of early stage AMD

How to Use the Amsler Grid Effectively

To ensure accurate self-monitoring, follow these tips when using the Amsler Grid:

- **Positioning:** Hold the grid approximately 28 to 30 cm (about 12 inches) from your eyes in a well-lit environment. Wear your regular reading glasses or your best-corrected near vision prescription.
- **Test One Eye at a Time:** Cover one eye to test the other. If both eyes remain open, changes in one may be masked by the stronger or unaffected eye.
- **Focus on the Center Dot:** Keep your gaze fixed on the center. Try not to let your eyes wander, as this reduces the effectiveness of the test.
- **What to Observe:**
    - Are all four corners and four sides of the square visible?
    - Do any areas appear missing, blurry, doubled, or distorted?
    - Are the lines straight, or do you notice any waviness?

If you observe any new visual changes or distortions compared to previous tests, mark the affected area on the grid and contact your retina specialist promptly. Consistent use of the Amsler grid can help detect changes early—before they become more serious or permanent.

What Do Changes to the Amsler Grid Mean?

Metamorphopsia. If you have dry macular degeneration or diabetic retinal disease, you may notice **distortion** of the central area (Image, above right.) This indicates a change to the macula in which the photoreceptors (light-sensitive neurons) have become displaced. This displacement could indicate the onset of the wet form of macular degeneration or diabetic macular edema.

Other pathologies that cause distortion: cystic macular edema and epiretinal membranes. This warrants additional testing by a specialist of retinal disease. Remember, early detection is key to the preservation of the central vision.

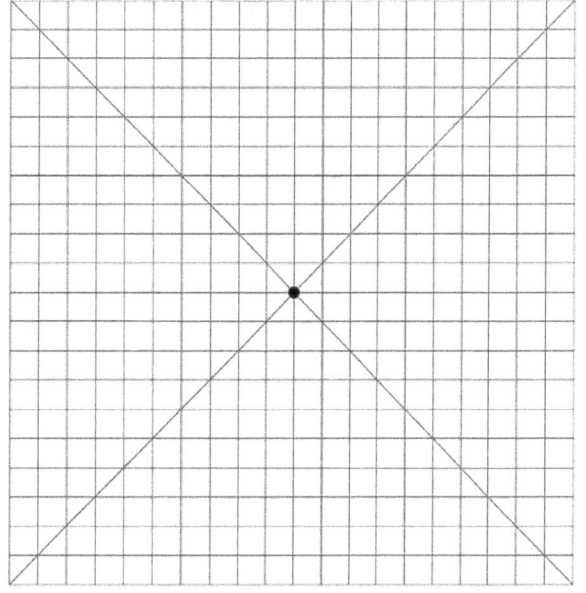

Missing or blurred areas. An area that is missing or blurred can indicate the presence of a scotoma. A **scotoma** is a blind area surrounded by normal areas and is caused by a degenerative disease. This blind area can occur in the central macular area. A scotoma of the central area will make it difficult to focus on the central dot of the grid. A grid with guidelines can help to find the central area to align the eye.

If the scotoma is in an area like the corner or one of the sides, it could indicate **visual field loss.** Visual field losses can indicate another disease process like retinitis pigmentosa, glaucoma, or pituitary tumor.

While the Amsler gird can be beneficial for detecting vision changes that otherwise might not be noticed, it is not perfect. It is not very sensitive. Room lighting, the distance the chart is held, and adequate near vision with a set of optimal reading glasses can determine if the test is effective in detecting macular changes. I have found the lack of patient compliance to also be a determining factor. Can't find it if you don't look.

Digital Tools for Monitoring Macular Degeneration

Is there an app for that? *Yes.*

Self-monitoring tools are not limited to printed Amsler grids. Today, a variety of digital options are available to help individuals monitor their vision at home. Amsler grid-based apps can be found in both the Apple App Store and Google Play—just type in "Amsler grid" to get started.

These self-monitoring apps generally fall into two categories:

1. **Independent Self-Monitoring Apps**
   These apps allow users to track their vision changes privately. Some include digital Amsler grids, reminders, and tools to document changes over time. While convenient, they do not share information directly with a healthcare provider unless the user does so manually.

2. **Apps Connected to Monitoring Services**
   Other apps are linked to subscription-based services that communicate with a participating eye care provider. These may offer more advanced features, such as personalized alerts, automated analysis, and the ability to send results directly to your optometrist, ophthalmologist, or retina specialist. Users must usually register and may need approval from their doctor to enroll.

Independent monitoring, apps that do not connect to an eye care provider required.

I reviewed several self-monitoring apps available in the Apple App Store. Google Play also offers a variety of options. Keep in mind that apps may change or become unavailable over time, so these are only examples available at the time of this writing.

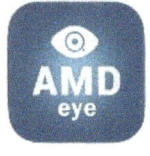

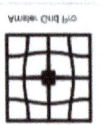

AMD Eye (*for iPhone, iPad*) This app was designed by an ophthalmologist. It is probably the most simplistic of the ones I tried. The grid does not have the standard 'square' appearance. There does not seem to be a way to mark up or keep a record of what is observed for future comparison. The user does have the capability to schedule daily or weekly alerts as reminders to test. There is also some macular degeneration education data on the app.

Amsler Grid Pro (*Google Play*) features interactive screens that simulate various visual distortions experienced by individuals with different eye conditions. The app offers multiple versions of the Amsler grid, including a standard free version supported by *ads* and anu in-app purchase for a premium package. Upgrading to the premium version enhances functionality, allowing users to track and monitor changes in their vision over time.

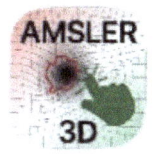

Amsler 3D

Medical

Amsler 3D. (*for iPad*) Uniquely, this app has an audio coach instructing the user on the correct testing procedure. It has several grid-type options including a flashing center dot option. The user has the ability to mark up the grid, label it with the date and save it under the setting indicated as *Reports*. The report can be emailed to a doctor or saved as a photo.

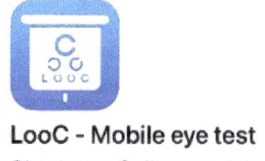

LooC - Mobile eye test

Check near & distance vision

LooC (*for iPhone, iPad*) This app uses an optotype called the **Landolt C** to test distance vision, near vision, color vision, and has an Amsler grid. It is interactive and uses an audio coach to give instructions. Results from the tests can be saved and shared.

MAVA: Mobile Acuity

Art Grichine

MAVA Mobile Acuity and Visual Assessment. (for iPhone, iPad) This is a very simple app, without options. The user can mark up the grid, identify which eye, and save and share it. That's it.

The app I am more likely to recommend to my patients is the Amsler 3D. I liked the audio coaching to remind the patient of the correct technique for testing and which large icon to tap next.

Apps connected to eye care professionals:

Some apps are designed to be used in partnership with an eye care professional. These typically involve more sophisticated tracking and secure data transmission.

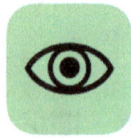

Alleye (for iPhone, iPad, Android) This app requires a recommendation by an eye care physician to access the app. The app should be installed at the eye doctor's office, where it can be demonstrated. The test does not use the familiar Amsler grid but does use an interactive task where the user moves dots into positions along a line. The test data is encrypted, transmitted, and stored by *Oculocare Medical.*

Alleye

OCULOCARE medical AG

OdySight. (Goole Play) This app uses gaming technology to engage users for self-monitoring between eye doctor visits. The developer warns that it requires some cognitive ability. It utilizes visual acuity and an Amsler grid.

OdySight

Monitor your vision from home.

While self-monitoring apps can offer a convenient way to track visual changes, especially for those comfortable with mobile technology, they may not be ideal for everyone. For individuals who prefer a more structured, clinically supported approach—or who need greater sensitivity in detecting subtle changes—there is another option. The **ForeseeHome device** provides an advanced home monitoring system designed specifically to detect ea0rly signs of progrssion in macular degeneration.

ForeseeHome Device for Self-Monitoring

ForeseeHome, developed by **Notal Vision**, is a home-based, tabletop monitoring device designed for individuals at risk of developing wet age-related macular degeneration. The test takes approximately three minutes per eye, and the results are automatically transmitted to Notal Vision for analysis. If any significant changes are detected, your eye care provider is promptly notified to arrange follow-up care—helping to ensure early treatment and preserve vision.

ForeseeHome tabletop monitor:

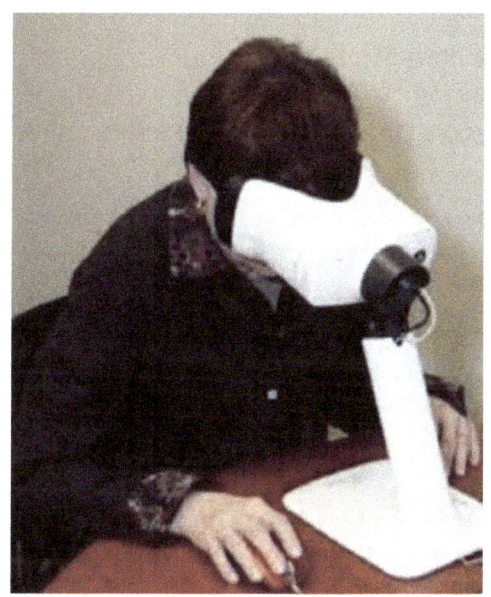

ForeseeHome addresses many of the limitations of traditional self-monitoring methods like the Amsler grid. It offers a more interactive and standardized approach, removing variables such as lighting conditions, head positioning, and eyeglass prescriptions. Unlike Amsler testing, the ForeseeHome testing ensures that your results are reviewed by a professional monitoring service, increasing both reliability and accountability.

The device is specifically designed to detect **metamorphopsia**—visual distortions that may indicate the development of wet AMD. It is best suited for individuals with relatively stable central vision and good cognitive function.

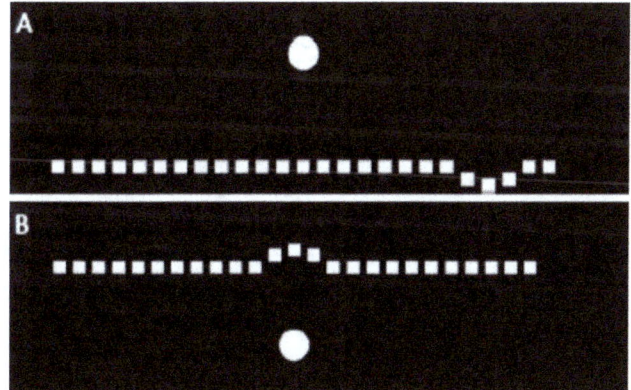

ForeseeHome test screen

Getting Started with ForeseeHome

To be eligible for ForeseeHome, your doctor must first determine that you're at risk of progressing to wet AMD. This is also the first step toward qualifying for insurance coverage—**Medicare** *may* cover *part* of the cost.

The setup process is simple. You don't need a computer, internet connection, or Wi-Fi. Notal Vision provides phone support to help you get started.

To learn more or find participating eye care providers in your area, visit the **Notal Vision ForeseeHome** website or use a search engine to locate their homepage. You can also contact Notal Vision directly to find doctors in your region who participate in the program.

In the End...

Self-monitoring empowers individuals at risk for progressive eye disease to detect subtle changes in vision that might otherwise go unnoticed. It serves as a valuable tool between comprehensive eye examinations—but it is not a substitute for regular professional care.

The traditional paper Amsler grid has been in use for more than a century. Its long-standing use underscores the importance of self-monitoring for the early detection of central retinal disease. It remains inexpensive, easy to use, and requires little training.

However, the Amsler grid is far from perfect. Modern digital apps and home monitoring devices offer interactive features, the ability to store results, and options to share data with care providers. These technologies may encourage more consistent monitoring. Yet they also pose challenges: not all older adults have access to digital devices, the confidence to use them, or the physical and cognitive ability to manage new technology.

Understanding the Genetic Side of AMD

Individuals diagnosed with mild to intermediate macular degeneration may benefit from genetic testing to help assess their risk of progressing to the advanced, vision-threatening form of the condition.

Patients often ask, *"My mother had macular degeneration. Is it hereditary? Will I get it too? What should I do?"* These are thoughtful and important questions. So, let's explore what we currently understand about the genetic factors behind this disease.

Understanding Macular Degeneration: The Basics

The macula, situated at the central part of our retina, contains the highest concentration of light-sensitive neuro-receptors. This area demands the most energy, oxygen, and nutrients in the retina due to its specialized cells. Consequently, it is highly susceptible to factors that reduce these essential supplies, such as cardiovascular disease, diabetes, and poor nutrition. Lifestyle choices like diet and exposure to environmental toxins can also impact blood flow, oxygen levels, and nutrient delivery. A compromised macula is particularly vulnerable to environmental factors like UV light and smoking.

Lifestyle factors, including diet, smoking, and exposure to environmental toxins like UV light, can also impair blood flow and oxygen delivery to the retina. All of these can contribute to damage over time. Fortunately, many of these risk factors are within your control.

But the question remains:

What Role Do Genetics Play?

Research has shown that macular degeneration is not caused by a single gene. Instead, it's a complex, multifactorial disease involving a combination of genetic variants and environmental influences. Different individuals may have different genetic "profiles," which interact with lifestyle and health factors in varied ways. This complexity helps explain why AMD progresses differently from person to person—and why developing accurate genetic tests for AMD risk has been such a challenge. (1)

Among the many genetic variants studied, two stand out as consistently linked to AMD:

- **Complement Factor H (CFH)** on chromosome 1
- **Age-Related Maculopathy Susceptibility 2 (ARMS2/HTRA1)** on chromosome 10

These two gene regions have been repeatedly confirmed in research as major contributors to AMD risk. (2,3,4) Individuals who inherit certain variants in these genes have an elevated risk of developing advanced AMD—especially when environmental factors like smoking are also present.

A commonly used analogy is that having these genetic variants is like carrying a time bomb: it may remain inactive for years, but the risk of it going off increases with age and exposure to harmful lifestyle or environmental influences. This is part of why the condition is called *age-related* macular degeneration.

What is the Purpose of Macular Risk Testing?

The goal of macular risk testing is to predict which individuals with early or intermediate age-related macular degeneration (AMD) are more likely to progress to the advanced, vision-threatening stage of the disease. With this genetic insight, you and your doctor can make informed decisions—implementing dietary and lifestyle changes and establishing a more personalized monitoring plan.

Although genetic testing is **not yet considered standard practice** in AMD management, it is available. Importantly, even without genetic testing, managing modifiable risk factors—such as smoking, diet, and cardiovascular health—remains an effective strategy to slow disease progression.

Keep in mind that not all insurance plans, including Medicare, cover genetic testing for AMD. Coverage policies vary, so it's important to speak with your healthcare provider and your insurance or Medicare plan administrator to determine whether this type of testing is included in your benefits.

What Genetic Tests are Available?

Several genetic tests are currently available for age-related macular degeneration. These tests analyze specific genetic markers associated with AMD risk and progression, offering a more personalized understanding of the disease. While **not part of routine eye care,** they may be useful for individuals with early to intermediate AMD who are interested in genetic insight and personalized treatment strategies.

ArticDx Tests: Macula Risk® PGx and Vita Risk

— **Macula Risk® PGx** was developed to predict the risk and rate of AMD progression. It uses known genetic markers—such as variants in the CFH gene (linked to inflammation) and ARMS2/HTRA1 gene (associated with neovascular or "wet" AMD)—along with non-genetic risk factors to assess a person's likelihood of developing advanced AMD. This test is most useful for individuals diagnosed with early or intermediate stages of the disease.

— **Vita Risk** evaluates how an individual's genetic makeup may influence their response to the AREDS formulation, particularly its zinc content. Studies have shown that certain genetic profiles may not benefit—or could even be harmed—by zinc supplementation. This test helps guide whether the standard AREDS vitamin formula is appropriate or if an alternative should be considered. This is a clear example of how personalized medicine can inform treatment decisions. (5)

Visible Genomics: AMD Risk and Progression Tests

Visible Genomics provides two AMD genetic tests: one assesses the individual's risk of developing AMD, and the other evaluates the risk of progression to advanced disease. The company emphasizes early detection and tailored management strategies. While their methodology is proprietary, they focus on using genetic information to guide future monitoring and care. For more information, type into your browser: ***Visible Genomics***.

23andMe AMD Genetic Health Risk Report

As part of its Health + Ancestry Service, 23andMe offers an Age-Related Macular Degeneration Genetic Health Risk report. This report tells users whether they carry specific genetic variants associated with increased AMD risk. While it **does not assess progression or supplement response**, it may provide helpful background for patients interested in their genetic predisposition.

How is the Test Conducted?

Genetic testing for AMD is a simple, non-invasive procedure. Your eye care professional collects a cheek swab in the office and sends the sample to the testing lab—either **ArticDx** or **Visible Genomics**. Results are typically available in about four weeks.

For tests like **Macula Risk®** PGx, the lab analyzes genetic markers across 12 genes and incorporates non-genetic factors, such as smoking status, to assign a risk category from 1 to 5. Individuals in Categories 4 and 5 have the highest risk of progressing to advanced AMD. Other test providers may use different reporting formats.

These genetic services offer valuable insights for patients concerned about AMD, especially those looking to personalize their care. However, it's important to remember that genetic testing is *not considered standard of care* and may not be necessary for everyone. The hope is that a deeper understanding of the genetics behind eye diseases will eventually lead to more targeted prevention and treatment options.

Potential Role of Gene Therapy in Macular Degeneration

Gene therapy for macular degeneration is currently in the research and clinical trial phase. The underlying concept is to repair, replace, or remove defective genes within the cells of affected tissues—specifically, the retinal tissue involved in age-related macular degeneration. The process begins with identifying the defective gene in the diseased cells. Researchers then design a functional version of that gene to correct the genetic defect. (7,8)

A major challenge in gene therapy is how to deliver the replacement gene to the appropriate cells. This is typically accomplished using a vector, most often a modified virus. These viral vectors are engineered to carry the therapeutic gene instead of their original genetic material, thereby eliminating the risk of viral infection. (9)

Although the concept is straightforward, gene therapy is highly complex and has taken decades to develop. At present, gene therapy efforts are primarily focused on inherited retinal disorders—such as Stargardts disease, Best disease, Sorsby fundus dystrophy, and cone dystrophies—where the specific genetic mutations are known and involve a single gene. These are known as monogenic diseases. (10)

In contrast, AMD is a multifactorial disease influenced by a combination of genetic and environmental factors. While certain genes, such as CFH and ARMS2, are associated with increased **risk**, the full genetic landscape of AMD is not yet completely understood. Because of this complexity, gene therapy for AMD is not currently considered a realistic treatment option. However, as our understanding of AMD genetics deepens, future gene-based interventions may become more feasible.

In the End...

Genetic testing for macular degeneration can provide valuable insight into an individual's risk of progressing to advanced stages of the disease.

Although gene therapy remains in the research phase and is not yet a viable treatment for AMD, studying the genetics of inherited retinal diseases like Stargardt's Disease and Best's Disease offers promising clues for future therapies.

Ultimately, the decision to pursue genetic testing is best made in consultation with your eye care professional. While it is not yet a standard part of AMD management, it represents a proactive approach to assessing and managing risk. As research progresses, we look forward to new preventative tools and treatment strategies that may change the course of this vision-threatening condition.

References

1. DeAngelis MM, Owen LA, Morrison MA, Morgan DJ, Li M, Shakoor A, Vitale A, Iyengar S, Stambolian D, Kim IK, Farrer LA. Genetics of age-related macular degeneration (AMD). Hum Mol Genet. 2017 Aug 1;26(R1):R45-R50.

2. Seddon JM, Gensler G, Rosner B. C-reactive protein and CFH, ARMS2/HTRA1 gene variants are independently associated with risk of macular degeneration. Ophthalmology. 2010 Aug;117(8):1560-6. doi: 10.1016/j.ophtha.2009.11.020. Epub 2010 Mar 26. PMID: 20346514; PMCID: PMC3711558.

3. Deng Y, Qiao L, Du M, Qu C, Wan L, Li J, Huang L. Age-related macular degeneration: Epidemiology, genetics, pathophysiology, diagnosis, and targeted therapy. Genes Dis. 2021 Feb 27;9(1):62-79. doi: 10.1016/j.gendis.2021.02.009. PMID: 35005108; PMCID: PMC8720701.

4. Heesterbeek TJ, Lorés-Motta L, Hoyng CB, Lechanteur YTE, den Hollander AI. Risk factors for progression of age-related macular degeneration. Ophthalmic Physiol Opt. 2020 Mar;40(2):140-170. doi: 10.1111/opo.12675. Epub 2020 Feb 25. PMID: 32100327; PMCID: PMC7155063.

5. Seddon JM, Silver RE, Rosner B. Response to AREDS supplements according to genetic factors: survival analysis approach using the eye as the unit of analysis. Br J Ophthalmol. 2016 Dec;100(12):1731-1737. doi: 10.1136/bjophthalmol-2016-308624. Epub 2016 Jul 28. PMID: 27471039; PMCID: PMC6570490.

6. van Lookeren Campagne M, Strauss EC, Yaspan BL. Age-related macular degeneration: Complement in action. Immunobiology. 2016 Jun;221(6):733-9. doi: 10.1016/j.imbio.2015.11.007. Epub 2015 Dec 19. PMID: 26742632.

7. Khanani AM, Thomas MJ, Aziz AA, Weng CY, Danzig CJ, Yiu G, Kiss S, Waheed NK, Kaiser PK. Review of gene therapies for age-related macular degeneration. Eye (Lond). 2022 Feb;36(2):303-311. doi: 10.1038/s41433-021-01842-1. Epub 2022 Jan 11. PMID: 35017696; PMCID: PMC8807824.

8. Jamil MU, Waheed NK. Gene therapy for geographic atrophy in age-related macular degeneration: current insights. Eye (Lond). 2025 Feb;39(2):274-283. doi: 10.1038/s41433-024-03463-w. Epub 2024 Nov 22. PMID: 39578546; PMCID: PMC11751089.

9. Nguyen, Khiem Sy BS, et al. Gene Therapy for Wet Age-related Macular Degeneration. Retinal Physician April 1, 2024 Vol 21, Issue Page(s).

10. Samiy N. Gene therapy for retinal diseases. J Ophthalmic Vis Res. 2014 Oct-Dec;9(4):506-9. doi: 10.4103/2008-322X.150831. PMID: 25709778

A Note from the Author

Thank you for choosing *Understanding and Coping with Vision Loss*. I hope the information and guidance in these pages have helped bring clarity to the many questions that can arise when vision begins to change. More importantly, I hope this book has reassured you that the experience of vision loss is shared by many people, and that with knowledge, support, and adaptation, it is possible to continue living a full and meaningful life.

If you found this book helpful, I would greatly appreciate it if you would consider leaving a review on Amazon. Your feedback not only helps other readers discover the book, but may also provide encouragement to someone who is searching for answers and support during a difficult time.

Thank you again for reading.

Terri Cyr, OD

Index